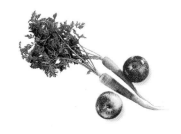

HEALTH AND HEALING
THE NATURAL WAY

EATING FOR
GOOD HEALTH

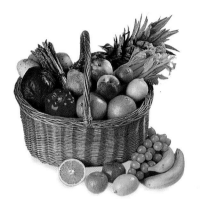

Health And Healing
The Natural Way

EATING FOR
GOOD HEALTH

Reader's Digest

THE READER'S DIGEST ASSOCIATION, INC.

PLEASANTVILLE, NEW YORK / MONTREAL

A Reader's Digest Book
Produced by
Carroll & Brown Limited, London

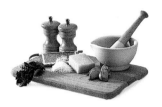

CARROLL & BROWN

Managing Editor Denis Kennedy
Art Director Chrissie Lloyd

Series Editor Arlene Sobel
Series Art Editor Johnny Pau

Editor Patricia Shine
Assistant Editor Melanie Halton

Art Editor Mercedes Morgan
Designer Michelle Tiley

Photographers David Murray, Jules Selmes

Production Lorraine Baird, Wendy Rogers,
Amanda Mackie

Computer Management John Clifford, Caroline Turner

CONSULTANTS

Prof. Tom Sanders, B.Sc., Ph.D.
Department of Nutrition & Dietetics
King's College, London

Moya de Wet, B.Sc. (Hons)
State Registered Dietitian

Paul A. Lachance, Ph.D.
Chairman, Department of Food Science
Rutgers University

MEDICAL ILLUSTRATIONS CONSULTANT

Dr. Frances Williams, M.B., B.C.h.i.r.,
M.R.C.P., D.T.M.& H.

CONTRIBUTORS

Dr. Lesley Hickin, M.B.,
B.S., B.Sc., D.R.C.O.G.,
M.R.C.G.P.

Roger Newman Turner
B.Ac., N.D., D.O., M.R.N.

Lyndel Costain, B.Sc.,
State Registered Dietitian

Anita Bean, B.Sc.

WRITERS

Anita Bean, Susan
Broadman, Helen Crawley,
Moya de Wet, Samar
El-Daher, Jeanette Ewin,
Miranda Holden, Judy
Marshel, William Murray,
Mark Ravenhill, Judy
Sadgrove, Roger Newman
Turner, Stephen Ulph

READER'S DIGEST

Series Editor Gayla Visalli
Project Editor Inge Dobelis
Senior Associate Art Editor Nancy Mace

READER'S DIGEST GENERAL BOOKS

Editor in Chief, U.S. General Books David Palmer
Managing Editor Christopher Cavanaugh
Editorial Director, health & medicine Wayne Kalyn
Design Director, health & medicine Barbara Rietschel

Address any comments about *Eating for Good Health* to
Editor in Chief, U.S. General Books, 260 Madison Avenue,
New York, NY 10016

You can also visit us on the World Wide Web at
http://www.readersdigest.com

Library of Congress Cataloging in Publication Data

Eating for good health.
        p.   cm. — (Health and healing the natural way)
    Includes index.
    ISBN 0-89577-832-7
    1. Nutrition. 2. Health. I. Reader's Digest Association.
II. Series.
RA784.E163   1995
613.2—dc20   95-8802

Printed in the United States of America
Second printing, July 1998

FOREWORD

The quality of your life—and how long you live—is to a great extent in your own hands. For what you choose to eat largely determines whether your body wards off or becomes vulnerable to a host of life-shortening diseases, such as cancer, stroke, hypertension, and heart disease. But changing to healthy eating habits, especially if you have not previously followed the guidelines recommended by nutritionists, can be a challenge. This is why EATING FOR GOOD HEALTH was created. Its goal is to provide you with clear, comprehensive, straightforward, and encouraging information that will enable you to change your diet from one that is potentially harmful to one that will help prevent disease and prolong life for you and your entire family.

This book shows you how to assess every aspect of your present diet and demonstrates clearly what is desirable in that diet. . .and what is not. It explains what protein, fats, carbohydrates, fiber, vitamins, and minerals are, which foods are their main sources, what their functions are in your body, and how much of them you actually need in order to maintain optimum health.

EATING FOR GOOD HEALTH also surveys the best diets worldwide so that you can choose elements from them that suit your whole family or the preferences of individual members. It clarifies issues of food growing and processing—from organic methods and use of pesticides to fortification, irradiation, and adding of preservatives—so that you can make informed choices. And it tells you how to choose the freshest and most healthful foods, then store, prepare, and cook them to obtain the best nutritional value.

Here is a very useful guide to selecting food that's best for your well-being and making dietary changes that will help you enjoy a long and healthy life.

CONTENTS

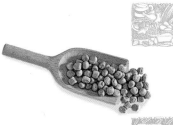

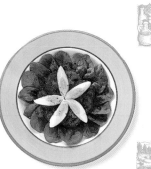
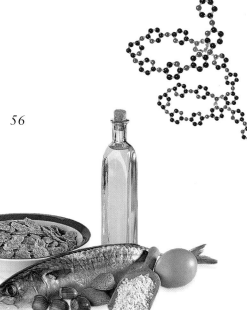

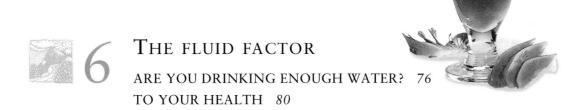

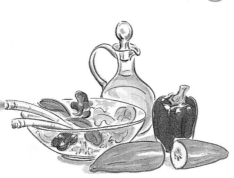

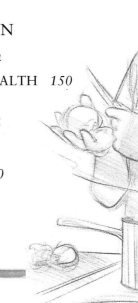

FOOD AND HEALTH —THE VITAL LINK

The alliance of modern chemistry with statistical surveys is leading to a new understanding of how what we eat affects both short- and long-term health.

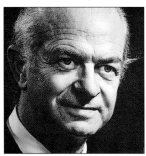

LINUS PAULING
American chemist Dr. Linus Pauling (1901–94) put forward the idea in 1970 of using vitamin C to cure the common cold. Since then, many studies have tested its validity but with little success. Yet research has shown that vitamin C does help the body to fight infection.

DISCOVERY OF VITAMINS
For centuries people suffered debilitating diseases, such as scurvy and beriberi, which are caused by vitamin deficiencies. When the first vitamin was recognized for its special properties in 1912, it was named A, and subsequent finds were named after the following letters of the alphabet.

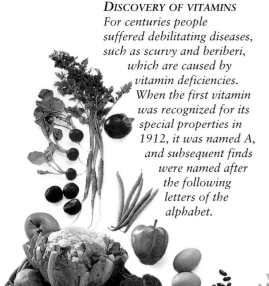

The body has a potent built-in alarm signal—hunger—to tell you when your supply of food, the "fuel for the body," is low and thereby ensure that you are never in serious danger of forgetting to eat. One of the most fascinating aspects of the way the body works is that this alarm signal is also choosy and at times asks for specific supplies, for example, sweet things when your blood sugar is low or water when you are thirsty.

What many people fail to recognize is that their bodies have more than just one signal. Tiredness, looking and feeling rundown, aches and pains, stress, even chronic disease—all these can be indications of a diet that is lacking in some crucial nutritional elements. But not all of these signals are instant or color-coded for easy reference, and that is the problem. Since no one sees or experiences the results of a poor diet immediately (often the effects take years to develop), few people realize how what they eat, as well as how much and how often, is important to good health. The old adage, "You are what you eat," has been scientifically proven. We now know for a fact that our diets affect the way we look and feel all through life.

A 20TH-CENTURY CONUNDRUM

Science over the past 100 years has made immense strides in medical knowledge and the treatment of illness, with the result that average life spans have gradually extended since the turn of the century. However, at the same time that a number of infectious diseases have been eradicated, and when technological advances in sanitation, immunization, bypass surgery, and genetic engineering are increasing life expectancies, the incidence of chronic disorders like cancer and heart disease has quietly shot up. It is even more incongruous that the main victims of these modern plagues live in Western industrialized countries, the very areas where medical research is most advanced and medical help most available.

Medical scientists are now quite certain that diet is a major factor in heart disease. The human body is not equipped to cope with the modern diet, which is often too high in saturated fat and too low in complex carbohydrates and fiber. Because insufficient food was, until modern times, mankind's greatest concern, the body developed the ability to make the best use of available seasonal supplies. It lay down fat in periods of plenty in order to survive during lean times. But today the main problem for most people in developed countries is excess rather than dearth, and the effects of this imbalance are proving to be equally dangerous. If diet is the cause of certain illnesses, however, it is fortunately also the cure.

THE NEW SCIENTIFIC CONSENSUS

Just a few years ago the idea that heart disease, osteoporosis, and cancer could be operated on in the kitchen was considered quackery. The discovery of wonder drugs and antibiotics after the Second World War brought a change in the way medicine was practiced and the body was perceived. As the achievements of laboratory medicine became ever more complex, treatment became concentrated in the hands of specialists who focused on specific aspects of the body. Pills and potions were seen as the real medicines, not herbs and other natural remedies. Nature, in the form of life's raw material—food—could not compete with the specialist's skills.

Once scientists discovered that the high-fiber, low-fat diet eaten in nonindustrialized countries seemed to give protection against certain chronic illnesses, the preventive powers of food and diet slowly came to be recognized once more. Certainly, changes in diets can save lives. Since 1967 deaths in the United States from coronary artery disease have fallen by more than 30 percent, in part because some people are eating fewer foods that contain saturated fat and cholesterol. But many people still do not know what food can do for them after it has suppressed hunger pangs. Old wives' tales about carrots helping you to see in the dark, spinach building up

A VEGETARIAN DIET
Many famous people throughout history have advocated a vegetarian diet. The Florentine painter Leonardo da Vinci (1452–1519), the American statesman and philosopher Benjamin Franklin (1706–90), the Irish dramatist George Bernard Shaw (1856–1950), and the Indian political leader Mahatma Gandhi (1869–1948) all abstained from eating meat. The reasons for becoming vegetarian may be religious, ethical, health related, or environmental.

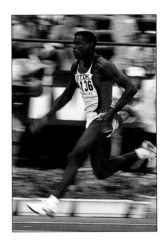

CARL LEWIS
The American track and field athlete Carl Lewis (b. 1961) follows a strict vegetarian diet. Lewis won four gold medals in the 1984 Olympics.

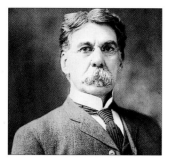

muscles, or fish sharpening your brains have proved not far wrong, and have triggered research leading to greater knowledge about the properties of food and the way your body uses it. The 100 trillion cells in your body undergo billions of chemical reactions every second; your health may depend on whether a particular enzyme or fatty acid is able to fulfill a needed function at the right moment. The foods you eat possess powerful capabilities to help and to harm.

ARE YOU KEEPING IN TOUCH WITH THE NEW FOOD FACTS?

Research into the health implications of food is advancing at a furious pace. Some findings are by now well known—that you should eat more fruits, vegetables, and whole grains and cut down on fat, for example. But do you know the latest findings that may be crucial to your health? For instance, do you know that eating oily fish helps to thin the blood and prevent clots? That garlic may have special anticancer properties? And what about the Food Pyramid? Do you understand the recommendations based on it?

The power of food to swing the balance of health one way or another is remarkable. Substances in some foods are toxic, such as the solanine found in sprouting potatoes. Other substances fight toxins, such as certain compounds found in cabbage that may help to combat the detrimental effects of air pollution on the body. Food has a particularly well-documented influence on heart disease. Some types of food may cause the buildup of plaque in the arteries, causing them to clog; other foods release substances that scrub the arteries clean. Saturated fat, for example, is the source for the synthesis of artery-clogging cholesterol in the liver, while the soluble fiber found in oat bran or beans, has been shown to bind intestinal cholesterol, thus helping the body to excrete it.

Foods can both promote cancer development and help to prevent it. Raw mushrooms, for example, contain hydrazines, and peanuts can carry aflatoxin from mold contamination—both of which are known carcinogens. Eaten regularly over a lifetime, substances in spinach, broccoli, and cauliflower have been linked to cancer prevention, as has an acid found in certain types of berries.

It is therefore not surprising that some medical conditions are treated through dietary changes. The treatment of gout prescribes fewer organ meats and less alcohol, and diabetes mellitus demands control of the carbohydrates consumed. There is scarcely a bodily process or disorder that is untouched in some way by what you put in your mouth.

INCREASING YOUR UNDERSTANDING OF FOOD

Every day seems to bring an avalanche of statistics and new diets to match them. A survey of English-language women's magazines not long ago showed that, on average, a new healthful or weight-loss diet was published in every third issue, only to be canceled out three issues later by one claiming to be more effective. Various foods can become the panacea or poison of the month. These dietary fads in turn subject the body to a total abstention from, or unusual concentrations of, selected foods. At times, food is granted second place altogether to vitamin pills and other nutritional supplements, in the belief that these may provide shortcuts to good nutrition.

But a miracle or fad diet is not the solution, neither are megadoses of vitamin pills. Instead, scientists now know that food and its effects are every bit as complex as our own bodies. Of the thousands of chemicals, minerals, and vitamins that exist in a single food, many are potential lifesavers or hazards to health, depending on how much is consumed over time. Here the old adage of variety being the spice of life is proving wiser than anyone ever knew. Eating different foods means that you are more likely to get a good supply of adequate nutrients, since something lacking in one food may be supplied in another.

The link between food and health is an everyday issue but also a complex one. So rather than trusting in food fads, you should learn how to balance your food intake. Small but well-informed changes to your diet will make a great difference to your sense of well-being.

EATING YOUR WAY TO GOOD HEALTH

The aim of EATING FOR GOOD HEALTH is to help you do just that— to think about the food you eat and ask yourself whether you are doing the sensible thing for yourself and your family. Based on the conviction that education is superior to following fashionable trends when making sound food choices, EATING FOR GOOD HEALTH leads you through the many layers of contemporary living where food occupies a key role—inside the body and in the kitchen, the laboratory, the factory, and the marketplace.

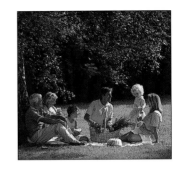

GENERATIONS OF
HEALTHY EATERS
The kinds of food you eat and how often you eat them have a major influence on your emotional and physical well-being. Much of the way people eat depends on habits fixed since childhood, but it is never too late to start a better diet. Whatever your age, you will always need a good supply of nutrients, and this is easily found in a well-balanced, varied diet.

"TO YOUR HEALTH!"
Drinking citrus-fruit juice will help you to increase your intake of vitamin C. A 6-oz glass of orange juice meets your daily need of this vitamin.

Chapter 1 will help you understand why good eating habits can keep you healthy. It contains guidelines for how often and how much to eat and how to identify the signs of nutritional imbalance. Chapters 2 through 5 explore how your body uses the essential nutrients: proteins, carbohydrates, fats, vitamins, and minerals. You will learn how much of these nutrients different foods contain and how to regulate and balance your nutritional intake. Chapter 2 also highlights the importance for vegetarians of combining plant foods to achieve a suffient intake of complete protein.

The body is even more sensitive to an imbalance in fluid than one in solid food. Chapter 6 details the body's requirements and evaluates the various types of fluid.

HEALTHY EATING FROM FARM TO TABLE

The past 40 years have seen a revolution for consumers, with the rise of new preservationand packaging methods and a reestablishing of organic farming. But the increased choices in packaging, processing, and farming techniques are in themselves no guarantee of a good diet. It is important, therefore, to be able to distinguish healthful foods from junk foods and foods that may be harmful. Chapter 7 provides detailed information to help you make well-informed choices.

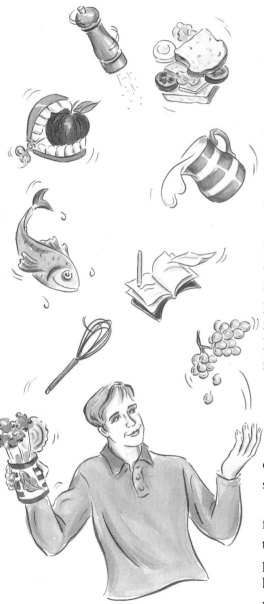

Chapter 8 evaluates diets from countries around the world and shows you how to take advantage of the Mediterranean, Japanese, and Chinese styles of eating. This chapter also explores the requirements of people with special dietary needs including toddlers, pregnant women, diabetics, and people with hypertension. By matching your diet to your lifestyle and developing better eating habits both at home and when you eat out, you can keep yourself in the best of health.

Chapter 9 tells you how to prepare foods for maximum nutritional value and stock up on the basics for a healthy diet. This chapter also conveys up-to-date information on long-term storage and preservation, refrigeration and thawing, and the optimum cooking methods for freshness, nutritional value, and safety from the perils of food poisoning.

EATING FOR GOOD HEALTH is designed to help you and your family understand more about the nature of the food you eat and the essential role of nutrition in the wider context of health—the promotion of physical and emotional well-being and the proper balancing of the social pleasures of the table with the vital requirements of the body.

ARE YOU EATING FOR GOOD HEALTH?

You may feel reasonably healthy and think that you are eating the right things, but statistics are saying otherwise. On a daily basis, the average North American eats just over half the amount of fruit and vegetables recommended by the World Health Organization and almost double the recommended intake of fat.

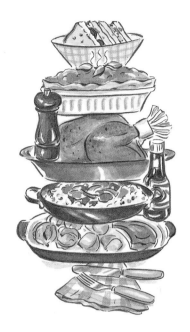

Q **HOW MANY MEALS DO YOU EAT DURING THE DAY?**
Do you usually eat one meal, two to three meals, or three or more meals a day? Eating one large feast a day is not very healthy. Nor is it any better to have a varying number of mealtimes from day to day. Your body works much better with a regular supply of nutrients provided in three or four regularly spaced meals a day. In particular, avoid skipping breakfast because you will expose yourself all the more to the temptation of sugary or fatty snacks, which you may crave by midmorning. Chapter 1 gives you some pointers on how to schedule your mealtimes.

Q **DO YOU EAT SNACKS BETWEEN MEALS?**
Do you always snack between meals, now and again, or never? In general, snacking is not a good habit to fall into if the snacks consist of sweets, chips, or other foods high in calories and fats. If you know that you do succumb frequently to the urge, make sure that your snacks will add something to your diet rather than undoing it. For more tips on healthy ways to snack, see chapter 8.

Q **HOW MANY SERVINGS OF FRUIT AND VEGETABLES DO YOU EAT EACH DAY?**
Do you have one, two, or the recommended five servings a day? The fiber in fruit and vegetables comes as an important extra to their food value. Provided your intake of essential proteins and fats is met, you would be hard put to eat too much fruit or too many vegetables. Some of the more sensational benefits of fruits and vegetables are listed in chapters 5 and 7.

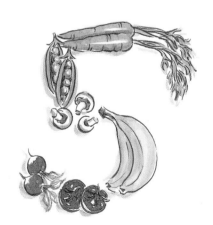

Q **HOW OFTEN DO YOU EAT CARBOHYDRATE FOODS WITH YOUR MEALS?**
Is it less, or more, than once a day? Complex-carbohydrate foods, such as bread, rice, potatoes, cereals, and pasta—particularly if unrefined—

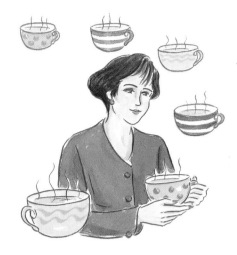

should make up at least half of your daily calorie intake. However, it's best to forgo high-calorie sauces on pasta and potatoes. The role of carbohydrates and ways of increasing the levels of fiber in your diet are discussed in chapter 3.

Q **HOW MANY CAFFEINE BEVERAGES DO YOU DRINK PER DAY?**

Do you have fewer than two caffeinated drinks a day, or from two to five? The benefit of caffeine is that it makes you alert, but this should be balanced by a moderation in its use, because caffeine can raise blood pressure. It is better to get out of the habit of using coffee and cola as all-purpose beverages and to drink them as little as possible. An evaluation of the advantages and disadvantages of caffeine are examined in chapter 6.

Q **HOW OFTEN DO YOU EAT RED MEAT?**

Do you consume red meat twice a week, more than twice a week, or every day? Red meats are high in saturated fat, but they are nutritionally important, so you should keep your consumption down to two meals with meat a week rather than eliminating it entirely. The value of meat and other rich sources of protein is illustrated in chapter 2, and chapter 4 details the types of fat that meats contain.

KEEPING A FOOD DIARY

Recording your daily intake of food and beverages is a very good way to monitor your present eating habits and to find out exactly what you eat. You may be asked to keep a food diary by a nutritionist, naturopath, dietitian, personal trainer, doctor, or other health professional. This will enable them to gain a more accurate picture of your eating habits, compare your intake with the recommended values for protein, carbohydrate, fat, vitamins, and minerals, and advise you on any changes you need to make.

When filling in your food diary, describe each food as accurately as possible; for example, a cheese sandwich may actually be three foods—bread, cheese, and mustard or mayonnaise. Give a clear description of the type of food, such as whether the bread is whole-grain, rye, or white; the milk is whole, low-fat, or skim; the spread is margarine, mayonnaise, or low-fat cream cheese. Include every spoonful of sugar in your coffee and every pat of butter on your bread.

FILLING IN YOUR FOOD DIARY
Write down everything you eat and drink for at least three consecutive days. Make sure that you include one weekend day. Take the diary with you if you eat away from home, for example, in the office cafeteria.

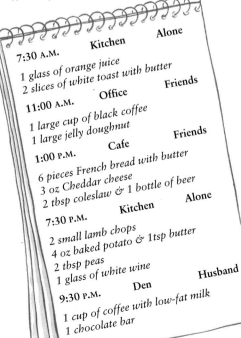

7:30 A.M. Kitchen — Alone
1 glass of orange juice
2 slices of white toast with butter

11:00 A.M. Office — Friends
1 large cup of black coffee
1 large jelly doughnut

1:00 P.M. Cafe — Friends
6 pieces French bread with butter
3 oz Cheddar cheese
2 tbsp coleslaw & 1 bottle of beer

7:30 P.M. Kitchen — Alone
2 small lamb chops
4 oz baked potato & 1tsp butter
2 tbsp peas
1 glass of white wine

9:30 P.M. Den — Husband
1 cup of coffee with low-fat milk
1 chocolate bar

CHAPTER 1

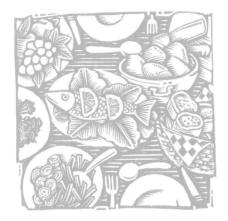

HEALTHY EATING

Not too many years ago, the optimal diet was said to be one high in quality protein, the kind found in meat and other animal foods. Today the advice is to cut down on red meat because of its high content of saturated fat. Moreover, experts advise, foods high in complex carbohydrates and fiber, such as whole-wheat pasta, whole-grain bread, and brown rice, should—along with plenty of fresh vegetables and fruits—form the largest part of a healthy diet.

ARE YOU EATING THE RIGHT FOODS?

Most people know that a well-balanced diet is vital for good health. Understanding your body's requirements and the foods that help meet them will enable you to make the right choices.

CHECKING LABELS
When choosing packaged products, read the labels carefully. Pay special attention to how much fat, sugar, and sodium (salt) the food contains.

Think of your body as a mechanism made up of billions of tiny chemical factories, linked in an endless process of utilizing energy, performing such functions as nerve transmission, and producing enzymes (body substances made from proteins that break down foods and regulate metabolism). Something as complex as the human body inevitably requires differing varieties and amounts of resources to function. Fortunately, everything the average healthy person needs is provided by a diet with the right amount of proteins, carbohydrates, fats, fiber, minerals, and vitamins.

THE BODY'S NEEDS

Proteins are the key building materials in all cells and are needed for growth and cell replacement or repair. Eating meat, fish, eggs, grains, beans, and dairy products will provide an ample supply of protein. From 10 to 15 percent of daily calories should be provided by protein.

Carbohydrates convert into glucose, the body's main source of fuel. They give you the energy to run a marathon as well as to sustain you during sleep. Even at rest, the body needs energy for growth and repairs.

There are two types of carbohydrate—simple and complex, or starch. The simple type, found in fruit, table sugar, and sugary foods such as cake and candy, are absorbed quickly into the bloodsteam and are either used up rapidly or stored as fat in your body. Starchy foods, such as pasta, beans, potatoes, and bread, take time to break down into the simpler sugar units that your body's cells burn for energy. As a result, a slower, steadier flow of energy is released into your blood, ready to meet your needs. From 50 to 60 percent of daily calories should come from complex carbohydrates.

Fats help form and maintain cell membranes, act as carriers for the fat-soluble vitamins A, D, E, and K, and are used in the production of certain hormones. They can

READING FOOD LABELS

Legislative bodies, recognizing that consumers need more information to make healthful choices, have passed laws in recent years to make product labels more meaningful. Manufacturers of processed foods in the European Community, United States, and Canada must now provide the following information on labels: the net weight or volume, a list of all ingredients, including additives, in order of weight, name and address of the manufacturer, and country of origin.

Manufacturers in the U.S. must also list the caloric value of one serving, suggested number of servings in a container and the total fat, saturated fat, carbohydrate, and protein contents, expressed in grams, as well as the percentage of daily value they represent based on a 2,000 calorie diet. Also included may be the potassium, sodium, cholesterol, or dietary fiber contents, plus the percentage of vitamins A and C, iron, and calcium, whether or not they are present in signifigant amounts.

also be stored in the body for future energy needs. Today, the recommendation is that no more than 30 percent of daily calories come from fat.

Fiber, or roughage, is the indigestible part of certain foods. It is important because, in combination with the water you drink and the complex carbohydrates you eat, it provides the bulk needed to carry waste products speedily from your body. Low-fiber diets are associated with constipation, hemorrhoids, colitis, and possibly even colon cancer. Good sources of fiber are cereals, grains, bran, fruits, and vegetables.

The trillions of cells in your body need minerals, such as iron, copper, zinc, sodium, calcium, and potassium, to carry out their essential biochemical activities. A diet containing a variety of foods is the best way to obtain a good mix of these minerals. Your body also requires other special food substances called vitamins. These are needed only in relatively small amounts but are essential components of a variety of functions. Vitamins release energy from food, help to make blood cells and hormones, and maintain healthy organs and systems such as the nervous system.

Finally, water is vital for life. As the principal component of body fluids it carries nutrients around the body, lubricates joints, and dissolves food for digestion and absorption. Water is contained in all the foods you eat and in the tea, coffee, milk, and fruit juice you drink, but you should also drink plenty of plain water each day.

How food is digested

The nutrients your body needs for energy, maintenance, and repair—including amino acids, glucose, fatty acids, vitamins, and minerals—must first be extracted from food by the process of digestion.

Digestion begins in your mouth as you chew food to break it up into smaller pieces. The food then passes through a long tube (pharynx and esophagus) that stretches down your throat and chest into the stomach. From there it goes through the small intestine (duodenum, jejunum, and ileum) and large intestine (cecum, colon, and rectum), exiting as waste product at the anus.

As food travels through the digestive tract, the salivary glands in the mouth and several organs —stomach, liver, pancreas, and intestines—add digestive juices and

MAKING THE RIGHT CHOICES

Different foods can provide similar nutrients. Most foods fall into one of four groupings, each of which provides a higher concentration of certain nutrients.

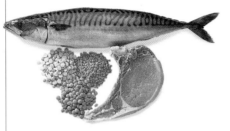

Meat, poultry, fish, nuts, eggs, and legumes (beans, peas, and lentils) are excellent sources of protein and also contain significant amounts of minerals and B vitamins.

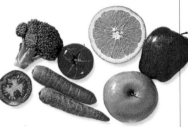

Whole-wheat cereals, breads, and pasta, brown rice, and potatoes are rich in complex carbohydrates, contain some protein, and are usually low in fats.

Dairy foods such as milk and low-fat cheese are excellent sources of quality protein, calcium, potassium, and B vitamins. Full-fat varieties or fortified dairy products contain vitamins A and D.

Fruits and vegetables are the best sources of fiber, minerals, and vitamins. You should eat a variety, as different vegetables and fruits contain different combinations of vitamins and minerals.

THE DIGESTIVE SYSTEM

As food travels through the system, it is broken down in various ways until all its nutritional value is absorbed. The remaining waste products are then expelled by the body.

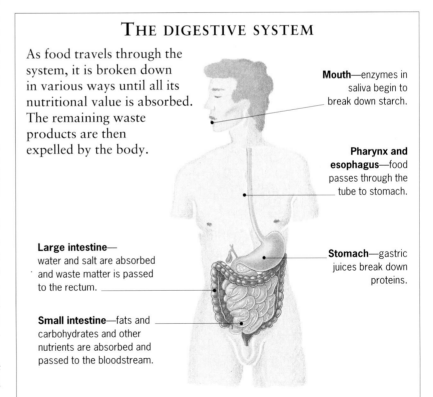

Mouth—enzymes in saliva begin to break down starch.

Pharynx and esophagus—food passes through the tube to stomach.

Stomach—gastric juices break down proteins.

Large intestine—water and salt are absorbed and waste matter is passed to the rectum.

Small intestine—fats and carbohydrates and other nutrients are absorbed and passed to the bloodstream.

THE FOOD GUIDE PYRAMID

In 1990, American government nutritionists developed the food pyramid to demonstrate how much food from the different groups needs to be eaten every day for a nutritionally balanced diet.

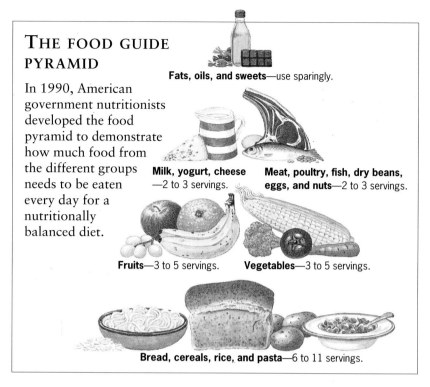

Fats, oils, and sweets—use sparingly.

Milk, yogurt, cheese—2 to 3 servings.

Meat, poultry, fish, dry beans, eggs, and nuts—2 to 3 servings.

Fruits—3 to 5 servings.

Vegetables—3 to 5 servings.

Bread, cereals, rice, and pasta—6 to 11 servings.

USING THE 12345 + FOOD PLAN
Australian nutritionists have developed an easy-to-remember food guide. For each day it suggests having one serving of meat or alternatives, such as dried beans, two servings of milk and milk products, three servings of fruits, four servings of vegetables, five servings of bread and other grain foods, plus a very small serving of whatever else you fancy.

other substances to help break down the food into simpler compounds. Once foods are digested, the smallest units of nutrients are absorbed through the linings of the digestive organs into the blood and lymphatic systems, which then distribute them throughout the body. The waste materials remaining after digestion is complete are expelled from the body as urine or feces.

BALANCING YOUR DIET

Doctors and nutrition experts tell us to eat a "balanced" diet, but this does not mean eating equal amounts of each type of food. You need to eat more of some foods than others to meet your body's needs.

For a balanced diet the foods you eat should work in harmony with one another. Over the years nutrition experts have drawn charts and plotted graphs to help people visualize which foods they should eat in larger or smaller quantities. As more has been learned about nutrition, the charts and graphs have changed accordingly. Once, the food groups were shown as sections in a pie chart; today the pyramid is a popular, more representative visual presenation.

Pathway to health

Many digestive disorders, such as indigestion, ulcers, and irritable bowel syndrome, may be aggravated by stress or deficiencies in the immune system. T'ai chi, the Chinese movement and meditation therapy, is thought to both cure and prevent such problems, especially stress. T'ai chi may also enhance the efficiency of the immune system by increasing the rate and flow of lymphatic fluid.

Pregnant women, nursing mothers, children, the elderly, and people who are ill may require somewhat different proportions of food, but for most people the pyramid guidelines are generally appropriate for a well-balanced diet.

The foundation of the pyramid is composed of complex-carbohydrates—cereals, rice, bread, and pasta. The greatest number of servings in your daily diet should be of these foods. Bear in mind, however, that the whole-grain forms are the best choices and are more healthful yet if served with just a little butter or a minimal amount of rich sauces, because these add calories.

The next level of the pyramid includes vegetables and fruits. Vegetables are most nutritious when eaten raw or lightly cooked. Six to ten servings of fruits and vegetables provide a wide array of vitamins and minerals as well as dietary fiber.

Meat and such dairy products as cheese and yogurt are important sources of proteins, and to two to three small servings each day are adequate. They are often high in fat, however, so you should choose leaner cuts of meat and low-fat or nonfat dairy products as much as possible.

The higher the fat content of foods, the less you need of them. Fats appear at the top of the food pyramid as a way of demonstrating how little you should eat each day. Products high in refined sugars also appear at the top, indicating that they are desirable only as a very small part of your diet.

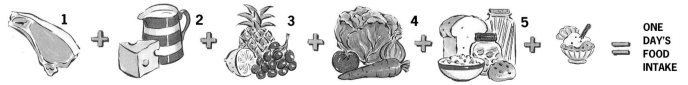

1 + 2 + 3 + 4 + 5 + = **ONE DAY'S FOOD INTAKE**

What is a portion of food?

Being able to judge adequate food portions, or serving sizes, is an important part of controlling your weight and maintaining a balanced diet. The portions listed in diet books and nutrition guides usually weigh between 3 and 3½ ounces. Sometimes food portions are listed in tablespoonfuls (tbsp), with 1 tablespoon equal to ½ ounce.

To improve your recognition of food portions, take a dinner plate similar to the one you use every day and, using a kitchen scale, measuring cup, and a tablespoon, portion out different foods. Look at how much space each serving fills on your plate. You may discover that your food likes and dislikes affect the size you think a portion should be.

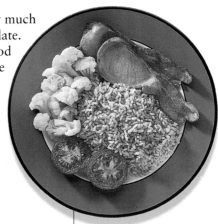

RECOGNIZING FOOD PORTIONS
Each of these foods is a portion: ½ cup of cauliflower, a medium-size tomato, ½ cup of cooked rice, and two strips of bacon.

COMMON FOOD PORTIONS

DAIRY PRODUCTS	WEIGHT	CALORIES	PROTEIN (in grams)	FAT (in grams)	CARBOHYDRATE (in grams)
Cheddar cheese	1 oz	114	7.0	9.0	Trace
Yogurt (low-fat) fruit-flavored	1 cup	231	10.0	2.5	43.0
Yogurt (low-fat) plain	1 cup	144	12.0	3.5	16.0
CEREALS					
Bread, whole wheat	2 slices	123	5.0	2.0	23.0
Roll, whole wheat	1 roll	90	3.5	1.0	18.0
Cornflakes	1 oz	110	2.3	Trace	24.0
MEAT					
Roast lamb, loin, lean	3 oz	171	23.0	8.3	0
Hamburger, lean, broiled	3 oz	231	21.0	15.0	0
Roast turkey, light meat, no skin	3 oz	133	25.0	2.7	0
Roast beef, lean	3 oz	189	26.0	8.7	0
Roast pork, loin, lean	3 oz	204	24.0	11.0	0
FISH					
Sardines, canned in oil	3 oz	177	21.0	9.8	0
Rainbow trout, baked	3 oz	128	22.0	3.7	0
Haddock, baked	3 oz	95	21.0	0.8	0
Salmon, Coho, poached	3 oz	157	23.0	6.0	0
FRUITS					
Apple	1 med	81	Trace	0.5	21.0
Banana	1 med	105	1.2	0.6	27.0
Pear, fresh	1 med	98	0.6	0.7	25.0
Pears, canned in heavy syrup	½ cup	95	0.3	Trace	24.0
VEGETABLES—RAW					
Broccoli	½ cup	12	1.3	Trace	2.3
Cabbage	½ cup	11	0.5	Trace	2.4
Carrots	½ cup	46	1.0	Trace	11.0
Cauliflower	½ cup	13	1.0	Trace	2.6
Spinach	½ cup	6	0.8	Trace	1.0
VEGETABLES—BOILED					
Broccoli	½ cup	22	2.3	Trace	3.9
Cabbage	½ cup	15	0.7	Trace	3.5
Carrots	½ cup	54	1.3	Trace	12.6
Cauliflower	½ cup	14	1.1	Trace	2.6
Spinach	½ cup	29	3.2	Trace	5.5

Hidden extras

When helping yourself to food, try to remember that equal-sized portions do not contain the same quantity of food energy. The number of calories in a 4-ounce portion of french fries (275) and the calories in a similar portion of spinach (24) are very different.

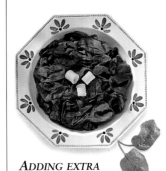

ADDING EXTRA CALORIES
Spinach is low in calories, but adding butter raises its calorie count substantially. Calories listed for a portion do not include toppings. For example, a portion of meatballs does not include sauce.

The Nutritionist

Nutritionists ask people about their eating patterns and other aspects of their lives and then advise them on how they can modify their diet to achieve better health, or make improvements to help treat a medical condition.

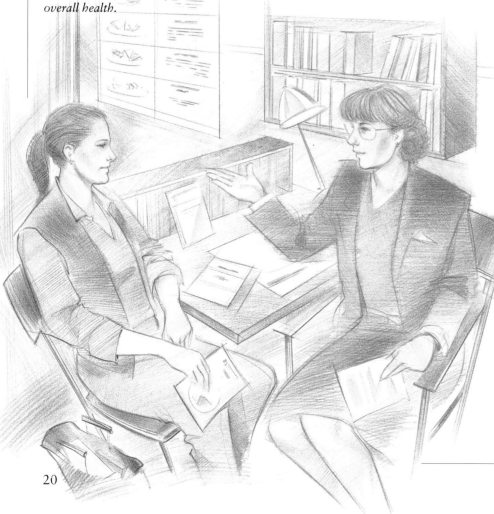

NATURAL GOODNESS
In line with current dietary guidelines, nutritionists recommend that you eat at least five servings of fruits and vegetables a day.

CONSULTING A NUTRITIONIST
Many people see nutritionists to get advice about a medical condition, for example, diabetes. Others may simply want to eat better to improve their overall health.

Consulting a nutritionist can be very helpful to anyone with dietary concerns. The nutritionist may be a medical doctor with training in nutrition, a PhD who specializes in nutrition, or a registered dietitian (see page 136). Ideally, a nutritionist should be a member of The American Society of Clinical Nutrition or the American Nutritionists Association, or be certified by the American Board of Nutrition. Credentials are important, because many states have no training or certification requirements for nutritionists, and anyone can hang up a shingle and charge for advice.

What happens on the first visit?
A nutritionist will ask you about your objectives (for example, to treat a particular complaint such as heart disease or to lose weight), your health, and your current diet. She will discuss your lifestyle, eating patterns, any allergies you may have, and any restrictions that you have placed on your diet—if you are a committed vegetarian, for instance. She may also ask you about any digestive problems and about your likes and dislikes concerning food.

If the aim is to lose or gain weight, the nutritionist may record your weight, percentage of body fat, and measurements (chest, waist, and hips). You will probably be asked to keep a food diary for a few days after your first session. This will be discussed on your next visit.

What value does a food diary have?
A food diary is the best way to find out what you are really taking in. In keeping this record, you write down the exact amounts of everything you eat and drink for three to seven days, including every cup of coffee and all snacks.

Using the completed diary, a nutritionist will be able to analyze your diet, compare your intake with the recommended values, check for any deficiencies, and then advise you on specific changes you should make.

Does a nutritionist do any tests?

If your diet lacks a particular nutrient and a nutritionist suspects that you are suffering deficiency symptoms, she will consult with your doctor. The nutritionist will describe the deficiency and suggest that you have a test—for example, a blood workup to look for anemia, which might be caused by lack of iron or vitamin B_{12} in your diet.

Will a nutritionist recommend recipe ideas?

Yes. Your food diary will reveal whether your diet is unbalanced or you have erratic eating habits. If the diary indicates you are often too busy to prepare proper meals—you may skip breakfast and eat too many snack meals—the nutritionist will suggest quick, nourishing recipes that include foods you enjoy and that you can prepare at home.

A nutritionist will check your food diary for sources of iron and how often you eat them. If there is a deficiency, she will give you recipes that include iron-rich foods, such as dark green leafy vegetables, meat, fortified cereals, and egg yolks. The nutritionist will also tell you how to mix iron-rich foods with foods rich in vitamin C to increase iron absorption—for example, by eating your breakfast cereal with fresh strawberries.

If you are a vegetarian, the nutritionist will suggest various ways of mixing beans and grains and other foods to get the right balance of amino acids.

How soon will my new eating habits have an effect on the way I look and feel?

The results will depend on what sort of changes you need to make and how soon you can put them into practice. Most people start to feel and see an improvement in two or three weeks. If you are aiming to lose weight, you should lose between one and two pounds per week—any more may be dangerous to your health—and therefore see a noticeable difference within a few weeks.

LOW-FAT COOKING

The recipe below was recommended by a nutritionist who believes that it is possible to satisfy a sweet tooth without indulging in excessive sugar and fat. This cake also happens to be quick and easy to prepare.

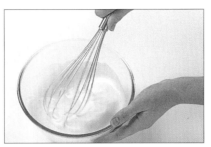

1 *Whisk 3 eggs and 1½ oz (3 tbsp) sugar until thick. Fold in 2½ oz (½ cup plus 2 tbsp) sifted flour. Fold in 1 tbsp skim milk and 1 tsp grated lemon rind. Spoon batter into a 7- or 8-in round cake pan. Bake at 350°F for 20 minutes or until cake springs back when lightly touched.*

2 *Let cool. Slice in half and fill with low-fat yogurt and fruit. Spread yogurt and fruit on top.*

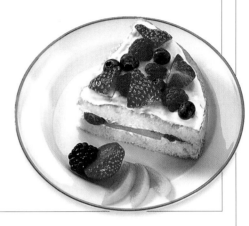

How many times do nutritionists see their patients?

Sometimes a single visit is sufficient to discuss the patient's main problems and provide enough advice to achieve the nutritional goals. At least one or two follow-up consultations may be needed to monitor progress and set further targets. Seeing the nutritionist more than once will help to keep you motivated.

WHAT YOU CAN DO AT HOME

To motivate yourself, write down all of your nutritional objectives. For example, "I want to feel more energetic and healthy" or "I want to lose seven pounds." Also keep a diary of everything you eat and drink for at least three days (see page 14 for details). Analyze your food diary to determine your good and bad eating habits.

▶ *Look at the timing of your meals. Do you eat breakfast? Do you eat at regular intervals during the day? Do you skip meals? These are important questions. Do you eat very little during the day but a very big meal in the evening? This eating pattern is far from ideal.*

▶ *Look at what kinds and amounts of food you eat. Eating large quantities of high-fat foods—for example, pastries and fried potatoes—is undesirable, whereas eating at least five portions of fruits and vegetables a day is good.*

▶ *Then look at the way your diet is balanced. Eating the same foods day after day is not as good for you as eating a wide variety of foods.*

▶ *Write down some easy changes you can make. For instance, start eating breakfast regularly. Do not skip meals. Eat fruit instead of cookies. Aim to make just one change at a time.*

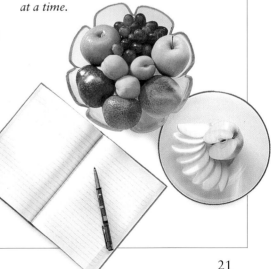

KEEPING YOUR BODY FUELED

Regardless of physical activity, your body uses up to 70 percent of its daily energy expenditure simply by keeping organs working, replacing cells, repairing damage, and building tissue.

Are snacks harmful?
Sometimes a snack is what you need to keep your energy level up, but it should be factored into your total diet. Consider the number of calories and amount of fat when you choose nibbles.

Snack foods such as potato chips, french fries, and nuts all contain high amounts of fat and are high in calories. Eat them only occasionally. For a more healthful snack, choose fruit, graham crackers, or perhaps some fresh vegetables with a low-fat dip.

Foods have different energy, or caloric, values because they contain different combinations and varying amounts of protein, fat, and carbohydrates.

MEASURING FOOD ENERGY
When food is oxidized, or burned, the energy, or heat, that it produces is measured in units called calories. Nutritionists actually measure food energy in kilocalories (1,000 of these units), but in popular usage the "kilo" has been dropped. The accepted international unit of energy is the joule (1 calorie equals 4.18 joules).

The basic nutrients in food—carbohydrates, protein, and fat—differ in the amount of energy that they supply. A gram of either pure carbohydrate or pure protein contains 4 calories; a gram of pure fat, however, contains 9, or more than twice as many. The other elements in food, water and fiber, supply no energy. This is why, for example, a 1¾-ounce serving of cauliflower, which is high in fiber and water, will supply only 7 calories, whereas a whole-wheat roll of the same weight will provide 135.

Everybody needs a certain amount of energy from food simply to maintain basic bodily functions such as breathing, blood circulation, and body temperature when the body is at rest. This is called the basal metabolic rate, or BMR. Further calories are necessary for activities. The number of calories each individual requires varies, depending on age, sex, size, metabolic rate, and activity. For example, a sedentary woman, 65 years of age, weighing 120 pounds, burns about 1,500 calories a day; an active 25-year-old woman of the same weight requires about 2,000 calories.

At certain times a person's basal metabolic rate may change, and affect calorie needs. During periods of illness or stress, the BMR tends to slow down and fewer calories are expended, but during pregnancy and while breast-feeding, it speeds up. A pregnant woman needs about 300 calories more a day, a nursing mother an extra 500 calories.

FOODS CONTAINING APPROXIMATELY 1,000 CALORIES

2½ bars of dark chocolate (2.8 oz each)
6 packets of peanuts (1 oz each)
4 cups baked beans (36 oz)
5 regular portions fast-food french fries
4 sausages (4" x 1" x ⅛")
7 cans of regular cola (12 fl oz)
15 slices of white bread
8 glasses of wine (6 fl oz each)
12 glasses of skim milk (8 fl oz each)
10 bananas
21 slices of ham (1 oz each)
22 oz of chicken (white meat)
32 carrots
57 servings of lettuce (¼ head each)

WHICH IS MORE FATTENING?
The number of calories in food can vary enormously. Both 40 tomatoes and two ¼-pound cheeseburgers supply 1,000 calories.

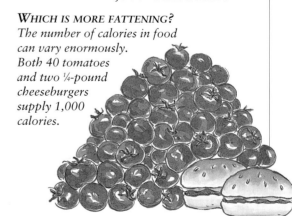

Active people use much more energy than sedentary individuals. Walking and gardening are some common activities that increase your body's energy needs. A man who drives to work, has a sedentary job, and spends most of his leisure time watching television will need only 2,400 to 2,500 calories, while an athlete in training will burn up 4,000 to 5,000 calories per day.

MAINTAINING BODY WEIGHT

Balancing the amount of energy you consume with the amount you expend is vital if you want to maintain your ideal body weight. When your diet is providing more calories than are being burned by your daily activities, the remainder will be stored by your body as fat, which may lead to obesity. But if your food intake is not fulfilling your energy requirements, your body will turn to any fat stored in tissues. If that becomes depleted it will begin to break down muscle tissue, including cardiac muscle.

Your scale is the quickest indicator of whether you are eating too much or just enough. But it's also useful to know about how many calories you normally burn in a day, so that you can match your caloric intake with your needs. To figure this out, first calculate your BMR by multiplying your present weight by 10. (This is a rough figure; your doctor can arrange to have your BMR determined more accurately.) If you weigh 150 pounds, your BMR equals 1,500 calories. To determine how many additional calories you need for everyday activities such as working at a desk and cooking, multiply your BMR by 0.30. (Example: BMR = 1,500 calories x 0.30 = 450 calories, or 1,950 calories a day for normal activity.) Now, add the calories required for athletic pursuits (see box, page 25), and you know your approximate daily caloric need.

DO YOU NEED THREE MEALS A DAY?

How many meals you have each day depends on your activity level and personal preference. Some people feel that they function best on three basic meals with no snacks, others thrive on five or more small meals, spread throughout the day. There is evidence that the latter is better for maintaining blood sugar levels and thus keeping a steady level of energy. It may also prevent overeating due to excessive hunger.

AGE AND ENERGY REQUIREMENTS

A 5- or 6-year-old child requires about the same number of calories per day as his or her 75-year-old grandmother, despite the differences in their weight and size. This is because their bodies are using energy in different ways. The child needs a lot of energy for growth and development; the matured adult, however, is likely to be fairly inactive and needs the energy primarily for maintaining bodily processes.

AGE	ACTIVITY LEVELS	ENERGY REQUIRED
INFANT		
Less than 1 year		950
CHILD		
5–6 years		1,710
BOYS		
12–14 years		2,640
GIRLS		
12–14 years		2,150
MEN		
18–34 years	Sedentary	2,510
	Active	2,900
	Very Active	3,350
35–64 years	Sedentary	2,400
	Active	2,750
	Very Active	3,350
65–74 years	Sedentary	2,330
75+ years	Sedentary	2,100
WOMEN		
18–54 years	Sedentary	2,150
	Active	2,350
	Very Active	2,500
	Pregnant	2,500
	Breast-feeding	2,700
55–74 years	Sedentary	1,900
	Active	2,250
75+ years	Sedentary	1,680

It's also been suggested that eating a big breakfast, less lunch, and a very small supper will aid digestion, by allowing the digestive system to break down food during the active part of the day and thus giving you a steadier supply of energy.

Dietary imbalance

In the Western world diseases such as scurvy and beriberi, caused by acute dietary deficiencies, are rare these days. However, more subtle health problems can evolve from eating too much or too little of certain foods.

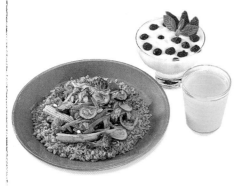

Feeling tired much of the time or suffering constant minor ailments can have many causes, including insufficient sleep, stress, and not getting enough exercise. If a checkup with your doctor reveals no underlying illness, your diet could be part of the problem.

Sugary foods, such as cakes and cookies or sweetened soft drinks, may produce a temporary sugar high, but then your energy level will drop dramatically. A diet heavy in such foods may also lack dietary fiber, which will lead to constipation and a feeling of lethargy. To maintain a steady energy level and stay regular, eat plenty of fruits, vegetables, and whole-grain cereals.

A lack of certain vitamins and minerals can also cause health problems. See far left column and box below.

FOODS TO PREVENT ANEMIA
Exhaustion and shortness of breath may be caused by anemia, a result of not getting enough iron. Animal foods, such as fish and red meat, are the best sources. Green vegetables and dried beans are good sources, too, but need to be coupled with foods rich in vitamin C (orange juice, for example) for better utilization of their iron content.

FOODS TO ALLEVIATE CONSTIPATION
An inability to pass stools can be the result of eating too little fiber. Unprocessed wheat bran makes feces bulkier and stimulates bowel function. But be sure to add fiber to your diet gradually; too much at one time can cause gas, bloating, and diahrrea.

CURING MINOR HEALTH PROBLEMS

Below are some common ailments that can be caused by an insufficient amount of certain nutrients. Eating more of the recommended foods should bring improvement in a few weeks. If a change in diet doesn't help, however, you should consult your doctor; these symptoms can also be indicators of other underlying disorders.

PROBLEM	POSSIBLE DEFICIENCY	EAT MORE
MOUTH		
Bleeding gums.	Vitamin C.	Citrus fruit, bell peppers, potatoes, brocolli.
Sore tongue, cracked corners, recurrent ulcers, cracked/dry lips.	Vitamins B$_{12}$, B$_2$, B$_6$, folic acid.	Yeast extract, potatoes, meat, poultry, milk, spinach, fortified cereal products.
SKIN		
Dry and rough skin.	Vitamins A, B$_2$, E, essential fatty acids.	Milk, dark green and orange vegetables, most vegetable oils, fish.
HAIR		
Poor growth, dry.	Vitamin A, zinc, essential fatty acids.	Milk, dark green and orange vegetables, oily fish.
NAILS		
Thinning; flattened and concave or spoon-shaped appearance.	Iron.	Red meat, fortified cereal products, kale, dried fruits such as dates and apricots.

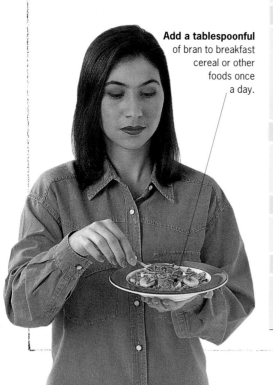

Add a tablespoonful of bran to breakfast cereal or other foods once a day.

Why breakfast is so important

While you sleep, your body is on a minifast, and blood sugar levels have become low. A breakfast that includes protein and complex carbohydrates, especially in the form of unrefined cereal or whole-grain bread, will recharge blood sugar levels and provide the energy you need until lunchtime.

Choosing a varied diet

Normally, during the course of the day, the foods people eat come from more than one food group. If you eat cereal and fruit for breakfast, soup and a sandwich for lunch, and fish or meat, rice, and vegetables for the main meal, you will have achieved a healthy and varied diet. But many people find it impossible to eat a balanced diet every day. Special occasions, vacations, illness, or pressures of work can all play havoc with mealtimes. However, studies have shown that it can be just as healthful to eat the right balance of foods over the course of three or four days, as on a daily basis. If you overindulge in fast food or chocolate one day, you can spend the next couple of days avoiding sugary desserts and following a diet that is low in fat and rich in grains, vegetables, and fruits.

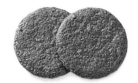

SATISFYING SNACK
Two whole-wheat crackers (1½ oz) provide 140 calories plus fiber.

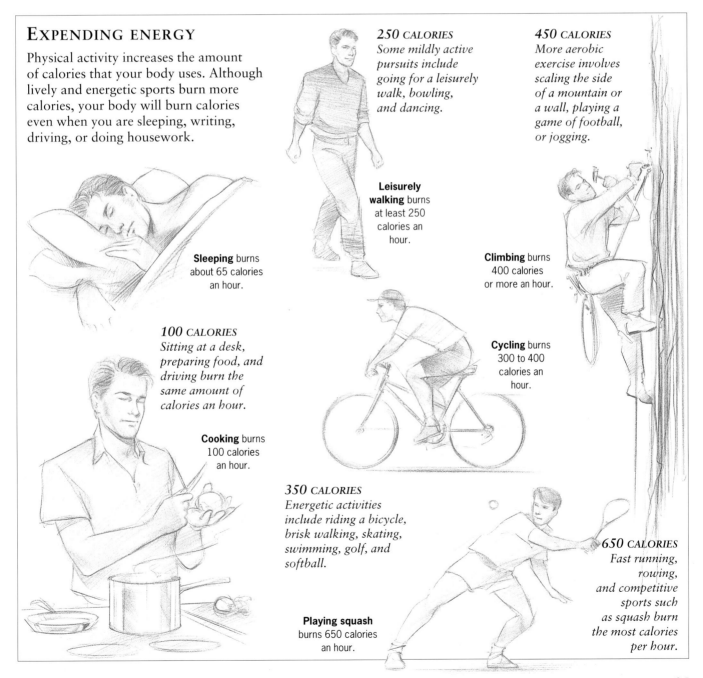

EXPENDING ENERGY

Physical activity increases the amount of calories that your body uses. Although lively and energetic sports burn more calories, your body will burn calories even when you are sleeping, writing, driving, or doing housework.

Sleeping burns about 65 calories an hour.

100 CALORIES
Sitting at a desk, preparing food, and driving burn the same amount of calories an hour.

Cooking burns 100 calories an hour.

250 CALORIES
Some mildly active pursuits include going for a leisurely walk, bowling, and dancing.

Leisurely walking burns at least 250 calories an hour.

350 CALORIES
Energetic activities include riding a bicycle, brisk walking, skating, swimming, golf, and softball.

Cycling burns 300 to 400 calories an hour.

Playing squash burns 650 calories an hour.

450 CALORIES
More aerobic exercise involves scaling the side of a mountain or a wall, playing a game of football, or jogging.

Climbing burns 400 calories or more an hour.

650 CALORIES
Fast running, rowing, and competitive sports such as squash burn the most calories per hour.

25

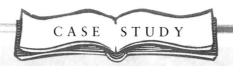
The Busy Family

Feeding a family is not easy. There are always the pressures of too little time, dissimilar food preferences, and the constant temptation to substitute less nutritious fast foods for better balanced home-cooked meals. The result can be a poor diet that causes health problems. The solution, however, does not mean sacrificing variety or favorite family meals.

Sandra Merton and her husband, Eddie, have two school-age children. In anticipation of college costs, Sandra took a job at a local nursing home six months ago, working the early morning shift. Since she started the job, she has noticed that the family's eating habits have become unhealthy.

Eleven-year-old Charlie eats nothing but hamburgers, french fries, colas, and sweets. He will not eat vegetables or, except for the occasional banana, fruit. Sandra suspects Charlie is not eating the breakfast she leaves for him. She is alarmed to see that he is developing acne. Fifteen-year-old Maggie tends to skip breakfast and eats as little as

possible at the table, although Sandra catches her taking snacks from the refrigerator while they watch television in the evening. Lately Maggie's hair has looked dull and dry. Both children have school meals, but the foods they choose are usually of the fast-food variety—pizzas, hamburgers, and tacos.

In order to help care for the children when Sandra is at work, Eddie switched to a night job. He is asleep when the children have breakfast but supervises the children's after-school activities. He shops for food when the refrigerator is empty, but his food choices are haphazard. Since they began their new schedule, Eddie has gained weight, which Sandra

believes is a result of his snacking on potato chips instead of eating a proper meal during the day. At work he buys a sandwich from the cafeteria and eats chocolate bars when he gets hungry.

During the week Sandra arrives home from work at two-thirty, and Eddie leaves at six in the evening. Sandra and the children eat their evening meal while watching television. Because her job makes her tired, Sandra often does not have the energy to cook, so they frequently rely on take-outs. The Mertons eat together only on the weekends, but the meals are quite stressful because while eating, Eddie and Sandra drill the children about their schoolwork.

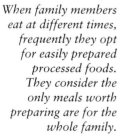

IRREGULAR HOURS
Shift work disrupts normal eating patterns and often means people feel hungry at times when a wholesome meal is not available.

SAVING TIME
When family members eat at different times, frequently they opt for easily prepared processed foods. They consider the only meals worth preparing are for the whole family.

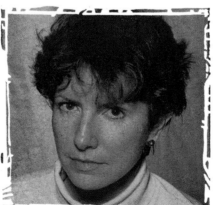

FINANCE
A diet of fast foods, snacks, and take-out meals is expensive, costing more than the same foods prepared at home.

HEALTH
Irregular eating habits create health problems because they make it difficult to achieve a balanced diet.

COMMUNICATION
Finding time to share ideas and information can be difficult for a busy family. When communication takes place only at mealtimes, tension and disagreements can make eating together stressful.

WHAT SHOULD THE MERTONS DO?

Sandra knows it is necessary to get every member of the family involved in changing their eating habits. Without cooperation little progress will be made and the eating situation will deteriorate further, harming everyone's health and appearance.

Since Saturday is a day when the family is free, Sandra should get them all together to discuss her concerns. Before the meeting she should make a list of the family's diet and health problems and how she thinks they can be solved. The family should agree to set aside one hour each week to discuss meal plans.

As a first step, Sandra should get everyone to take part in choosing the foods they eat, with an emphasis on good health.

Eddie must realize that he has to lose weight—he has gained 15 pounds since he started on the night shift. He has to abandon his unhealthy snacking habit, especially during the day. He should also investigate various forms of exercise that he can do during his free time.

Both children must alter their eating habits—Charlie to a less "high-fat and sugar" diet and Maggie to a diet that is much more balanced.

Meals need to be made into a more relaxed occasion, and discussions relating to schoolwork should be saved for another time.

Action Plan

IRREGULAR HOURS
Help Eddie make a list of tasty, healthful foods he can prepare for himself after he returns home from work and during the day. Substitute low-calorie snacks, such as fruit, for the chocolate eaten during the work shift.

FINANCE
Collect the bills for food purchased over a four-week period, and add up how much was spent on various items. Draft a food budget and an eating plan that provide a balanced diet—and are cheaper as well.

HEALTH
Make a list of all the health problems and conditions the family faces because of poor dietary habits. Also make a list of healthful foods that will help the family to avoid vitamin and mineral deficiencies. Begin looking for interesting ways to incorporate these items into the family's new eating plan.

COMMUNICATION
Reserve family mealtimes for listening to the children, and discuss pleasant and noncontroversial topics. Let the children have their say when shopping and cooking the family's meals. Having greater control will make them more interested in the foods they eat.

SAVING TIME
When preparing meals on the weekend, make extra and freeze in portion-size containers. (Portions of food can be microwaved quickly and easily when Eddie is by himself during the day; Sandra and the children can do the same later in the evening.)

HOW THINGS TURN OUT FOR THE MERTONS

The family meetings were successful for the first three weeks, and then the children became bored and restless, so discussions were cut down to 30 minutes.

Sandra and Eddie set a food budget for the month and a limit on take-out food to once a week. However, take-outs still figure in at least two dinners a week, and the budget has not yet been met. But substantial savings are being made, and these are being put aside for the college fund.

Eddie finds it hard to break his snack habit during the day, so every time he gets hungry he takes a brisk walk. When shopping for food, he tries to resist buying unhealthy snack fare; he now buys more fresh fruits and vegetables.

The Saturday shopping trip is being done on a rotation system, with either Maggie or Charlie accompanying one of the parents. This has made both children more food conscious, and this new awareness has carried over into their

school meals, which no longer consist solely of fast foods. With Charlie's help, Maggie has started to select recipes for her mother to make. She now devotes some of her time to reading about health and beauty in addition to pop stars.

After a month Sandra told everyone she wanted them to take turns making the evening meal. She knew the family had turned the corner when Charlie volunteered to prepare the meat loaf and potatoes for Sunday lunch.

THE EFFECTS OF CULTURE ON EATING

Many things besides availability and nutritional value affect choices of food. Some of them have to do with long-standing traditions, others with more subliminal influences.

Savoring the flavor
French children learn how to use their sense of taste in school. Part of their curriculum involves identifying and describing the tastes of saltiness, bitterness, sweetness, and sourness. This is followed by exercises in which food textures are explored. Finally, the children learn how to describe blends of flavors and consistencies in specific foods.

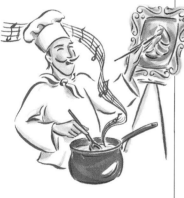

*REFINED TASTE
The French believe that, like a fine painting or a piece of classical music, the artistry of a cook and the quality of a meal may be appreciated fully only when the sense of taste has been educated.*

Much more than flavor and food values influence decisions about what to eat. Cultural background may make food that is well regarded in one country, for instance, horse meat in France, an anathema in others, such as the horse-loving United Kingdom.

Political beliefs occasionally alter eating habits. Low pay for and poor treatment of grape pickers on the West Coast of the United States spurred Cesar Chavez (1927–94) to lead a successful embargo of the fruit during the 1960's. Another aspect is religion. Many Jews and Muslims don't eat pork because the pig is regarded as unclean. (This prohibition may have had its origins in a caution about eating meat that can cause disease if undercooked.)

Subliminal desires

Food and drink manufacturers often use subtle means to persuade you to choose their products. For example, when watching movies and television dramas, if you see

THE "IDEAL" SHAPE
Fashion usually features models who are thin, because designers claim that clothes hang better on them. Many women regard this thinness as worthy of being emulated. In attempting to achieve this "ideal" body shape, they may come to regard all food as the enemy. In fact, food in the form of a well-balanced diet is the best friend your body has.

a certain brand of soda in the hero's hand, it probably is not there by chance. Companies pay a lot of money to advertise in this way—it is what the advertising industry calls product placement. Their hope is that the next time you buy a soft drink, the image you have seen, although it may not come to mind, may have had a subconscious influence on your choice of product.

SYMBOLISM, FESTIVALS, AND CELEBRATIONS

Food plays a prominent role in many of society's rituals, particularly festivals and celebrations, but even funerals. Food is often used as a sign of love and friendship. Sweets, for example, are associated with comfort and security; chocolates are given to friends and relatives as a sign of affection and are a particularly popular Valentine's Day gift.

Many foods are traditionally eaten at certain festivals and celebrations. Roast turkey and pumpkin pie, for example, are the menu features at Thanksgiving in the United States, whereas eggs symbolize Easter in many parts of the world.

Quite a few occasions are incomplete without a cake. Cakes are eaten at birthday parties, christenings, and weddings. The tiered cake is the focal point of most wedding celebrations, with the cutting of the cake being a time-honored tradition. A layer of wedding cake is often saved to be eaten on the first anniversary or at the christening of the couple's first baby.

CHAPTER 2

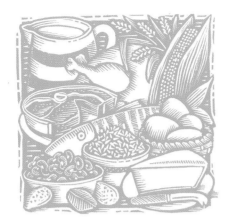

THE POWER OF PROTEIN

Proteins are essential constituents of all human cells, controlling such vital processes as metabolism and providing the structural basis of many body tissues, such as muscles and skin. They enable the body to grow and repair itself, and they play a role in protecting the body against infection. Protein-rich foods are mainly of animal origin—meat, fish, poultry, eggs, and milk. But some protein is also present in plant foods; good sources are wheat, rice, nuts, and legumes such as beans and lentils.

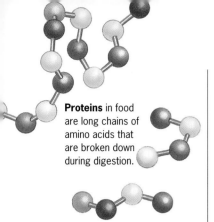

Proteins in food are long chains of amino acids that are broken down during digestion.

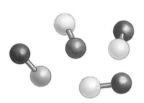

Polypeptides, which are the next stage in protein digestion, are shorter chains.

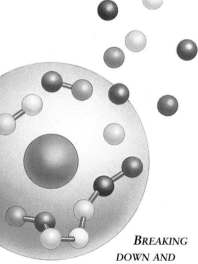

Peptides are chains with yet fewer links, which then break down into constituent amino acids.

Individual amino acids are finally reassembled into the new proteins that are needed by the body.

BREAKING DOWN AND REASSEMBLING PROTEIN
The proteins that are used by body cells differ from those found in foods, although both types consist of the same amino acids. After ingestion, the amino acids in foods are rearranged into the protein structures needed by the body.

PROTEIN FOR LIFE

Proteins, vital for growth or repair of every cell in the human body, are available in all our foods except sugar and oil. From 10 to 15 percent of daily calories should come from protein.

Proteins are the building blocks of life, playing a major role in thousands of the body's vital functions. Not only are they needed for the growth and repair of all cells, but also are involved in the production of enzymes used for digestion and metabolism, insulin and other hormones, chemicals that control our heredity, and the antibodies that protect us from disease. The proper functioning of memory and nerves is not be possible without proteins.

There are more than 50,000 different proteins in the body, all made up of chains of amino acids. Some of the amino acids are recycled from the body tissue that is being rebuilt; some must be supplied by dietary proteins, because the body constantly loses some protein through normal wear and tear. The body then synthesizes the new amino acids into proteins tailored for its various vital processes. Any dietary protein not needed for these functions is stored as fat. Some may also be converted to glucose and burned for energy.

Amino acids come in 20 different forms. Nine of them fall into the category termed essential, which means that they have to be supplied by food because the body is unable to manufacture them. Lack of even one essential amino acid over a period of time can cause you to lose muscle. The remaining 11 amino acids are called nonessential, because the body is able to synthesize them itself.

HOW THE BODY USES PROTEIN

The enzymes in the digestive system separate dietary protein into its constituent amino acids, which then circulate in the bloodstream. The body's cells, in turn, stack the amino acids up in the combinations that they need. Each amino acid has a

FOOD PROTEIN QUALITY

A food's protein quality is determined by the amounts of essential amino acids that it contains. Eggs are the best source of protein—they have a maximum score of 100. This chart shows the protein quality of foods as measured against the egg.

HIGH- AND LOW-QUALITY PROTEIN
Animal foods, such as fish and meat, provide the body with sufficient essential amino acids. Plant foods, on the other hand, lack one or more of the essential amino acids and therefore have a poor protein quality. When cereals and legumes are eaten together, however, they complement each other to provide a higher-quality—and more complete—protein.

PROTEIN SOURCE	PROTEIN QUALITY
Egg	100
Fish	90
Meat	80
Cow's milk	80
Grain with legumes	80
Soybeans	75
Oatmeal	65
Rice	57
Peas	48
Lentils	45
Kidney beans	44
Whole-grain bread	40

unique role, and another one cannot be used in its place. This is why a diet should be varied enough to provide all the amino acids that are needed.

COMPLETE AND INCOMPLETE PROTEINS

Proteins vary in the number, type, and arrangement of their amino acids, and this defines their quality, sometimes referred to as completeness or "biological value."

Animal foods are a major source of protein, and the protein present in meat, fish, eggs, milk, and milk products contains all the essential amino acids in the proportions the body requires. Animal protein, therefore, is known as "complete" protein.

The protein in plant foods—cereals (grain products), nuts, and legumes (peas, beans, and lentils)—also contributes different amounts and types of essential amino acids. However, unlike animal sources, no single plant source is able to provide a full complement of essential amino acids. Plant proteins, therefore, are "incomplete" and have a low biological value.

In order for plant foods to supply complete proteins, those that are low in certain essential amino acids should be eaten with those that are relatively high in those amino acids. Wheat, corn, and rice, for example, contain plenty of methionine but not very much lysine, whereas legumes contain a good supply of lysine but not much methionine. Without knowing the chemical and biological reasons, cooks around the world for centuries have combined grains and legumes to provide complete protein in a single dish—for example, rice and lentils, bulgur and kidney beans, or pinto beans with corn tortillas.

How much protein is enough?

The body gains and loses protein every day —for instance, simply cutting your nails or hair will cause a minor loss of protein, whereas every four days one-half of the intestinal lining, which has a vast surface area, is replaced. Therefore it is important to have some protein every day to replace the worn-out tissues that result from general bodily wear and tear and to manufacture new blood cells, hormones, and enzymes.

Bodily proteins

There are two distinct types of protein in the body—insoluble structural proteins, which are basically fibrous in form, and physiologically active soluble proteins, which have a globular structure.

The fibrous type includes such proteins as keratin in hair and nails; myosin in muscle tissue; collagen in connective tissues such as skin, tendons, and cartilage; and fibrin found in scar tissue.

The physiologically active class of protein includes most of the enzymes involved in the metabolic activities of the body. This type of protein also includes a number of hormones, for example, insulin and prolactin (milk secretion); hemoglobin, which transports oxygen in the blood; and the antibodies used in the body's defense system.

COMPLEMENTARY PROTEINS

Complementary protein food sources do not need to be eaten at the same meal, but they do need to be eaten at the next meal on the same day. This is because the body stores essential amino acids for only a few hours.

MATCHING YOUR PROTEIN FOODS
The solid red line in this diagram shows the better combination of plant foods to obtain quality protein. The broken green line shows the combination that does not always provide complete protein.

‒ ‒ ‒ **Weaker combination for obtaining complete protein**

——— **Good combination for obtaining complete protein**

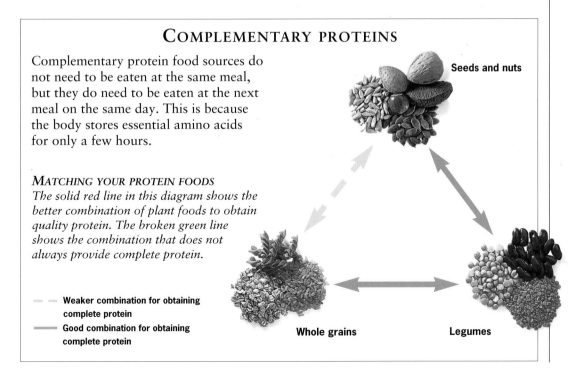

Seeds and nuts

Whole grains　　**Legumes**

RECOMMENDED DAILY INTAKE OF PROTEIN

The amount of protein you need will vary throughout your life. Pregnant women need an extra 10 grams of protein per day. Mothers who are breast-feeding need an extra 12 to 15 grams.

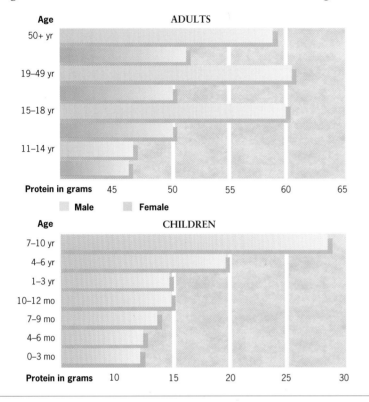

ADULTS

Age	
50+ yr	
19–49 yr	
15–18 yr	
11–14 yr	

Protein in grams 45 50 55 60 65

■ Male   ■ Female

CHILDREN

Age	
7–10 yr	
4–6 yr	
1–3 yr	
10–12 mo	
7–9 mo	
4–6 mo	
0–3 mo	

Protein in grams 10 15 20 25 30

An individual's protein requirements are often calculated according to body weight measured in kilograms. To convert your weight from pounds to kilograms, divide it by 2.2. Multiply that number by 0.8 to determine how many grams of protein, on average, you should have daily to maintain your health. For example, if you weigh 126 pounds, or 57 kilograms (126 divided by 2.2), your average daily protein requirement is 46 grams (57 x 0.8).

In a well-balanced diet between 10 and 15 percent of the total calories should come from protein. An average-size middle-aged man, for example, could easily fulfill his daily protein need with a cheese sandwich, a cup of milk, one serving of chicken breast, and one portion each of potatoes and peas. On the other hand, a woman in her sixties, who requires fewer calories, would need only 8 ounces of yogurt, an egg, a glass of milk, a small serving of fish, some rice, and three whole wheat crackers.

At various times in life people require extra protein. Pregnant and breast-feeding women must have an adequate intake for development of the fetus and production of milk (10 to 15 grams more than women who are not pregnant or lactating). People suffering from a severe injury, such as a

PICK A PORTION OF PROTEIN

Illustrated below are the amounts of protein in high-protein foods like meat, fish, and milk. Another food rich in complete protein is the egg (see page 30).

Also shown are the amounts of protein in plant foods. Because these amino acids are incomplete, they need to be complemented as shown on page 31.

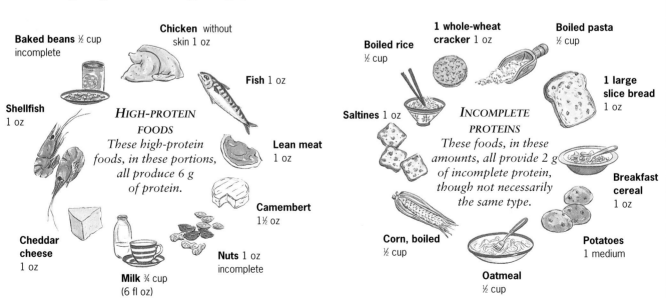

Baked beans ½ cup incomplete

Chicken without skin 1 oz

Fish 1 oz

Shellfish 1 oz

HIGH-PROTEIN FOODS
These high-protein foods, in these portions, all produce 6 g of protein.

Lean meat 1 oz

Camembert 1½ oz

Cheddar cheese 1 oz

Milk ¾ cup (6 fl oz)

Nuts 1 oz incomplete

Boiled rice ½ cup

1 whole-wheat cracker 1 oz

Boiled pasta ½ cup

Saltines 1 oz

INCOMPLETE PROTEINS
These foods, in these amounts, all provide 2 g of incomplete protein, though not necessarily the same type.

1 large slice bread 1 oz

Breakfast cereal 1 oz

Corn, boiled ½ cup

Potatoes 1 medium

Oatmeal ½ cup

THE KIDNEYS AND EXCESS PROTEIN

As part of the urinary tract, the kidneys have two main functions: filtering the blood and excreting waste products and excess water. The most important waste products are those generated by the breakdown of proteins. Proteins have a high nitrogen content, which is dangerous to the body, and this must be filtered out. If too many high-protein foods are eaten, the kidneys must work much harder to remove the waste matter. The increased level of urine that is needed to excrete the nitrogen puts a strain on the kidneys and may lead to renal disorders or damage to the kidneys' filtering units, the glomeruli. If the glomeruli are damaged, blood and protein will be lost in the urine. Mild versions of this condition occur naturally with age, but severe cases may ultimately lead to the destruction of the kidneys.

EXCRETING URINE
Excess amino acids that are not needed by the body are converted to urea in the liver. Urea travels via the bloodstream to the kidneys and is removed in urine.

Tubule—reabsorbs water, salt, and other essential substances such as amino acids.

Ureter—waste fluid (urine) passes into these tubes and is then excreted.

Glomeruli—each glomerulus acts as a filter for waste products.

Special needs
Broken bones and severe injury may cause significant loss of protein. A convalescent's diet should therefore be high in protein. If appetite is poor, offer fish, milk, eggs, and nuts, which are often more appealing than meats, and prepare dishes supplemented with powdered milk, soy flour, and dried yeast. Be sure also to provide adequate carbohydrates and fats to prevent the body using its supply of protein for energy.

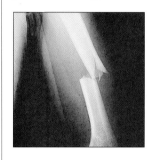

LOSING PROTEIN
About 60 grams of protein a day may be lost owing to injury.

broken limb, need to significantly increase their protein intake to help the body repair the damage. Children's protein requirements are also greater than those of adults, because their bodies are constantly laying down new tissue while they are growing. Even a month's deficiency may result in stunted growth and possibly impaired mental development. Prolonged protein deprivation can lead to death.

Too little protein can upset the body's fluid balance and lead to edema (fluid retention). The swollen stomachs of children in underdeveloped countries who suffer from kwashiorkor (protein malnutrition) are caused by fluid retention.

DID YOU KNOW?
The essential amino acid phenylalanine forms part of the artificial sweetener aspartame, which is used in a wide range of sugar-free foods and beverages, such as diet yogurt and low-calorie colas. Although aspartame is considered a safe product by government health departments, it should always be used in moderation.

How much protein is too much?
While too little protein is bad, eating too much also may be harmful. Excess protein, as much as 150 grams per day, or 300 percent of the daily requirement, can be consumed by eating a breakfast of a two-egg omelet made with ham and cheese, wholewheat toast and a glass of milk; a lunch of 3 ounces of turkey in a whole-wheat pita and a glass of milk; a snack of peanuts (1 oz); and a sirloin steak (6 oz) with baked potatoes, peas, a whole-wheat roll and frozen yogurt (1 cup) for dinner.

Such excessive amounts of protein place a strain on the kidneys. The body's tissues do not use the nitrogen portion of the protein molecule and it is excreted by the kidneys. The more protein consumed, the more fluid the kidneys need to flush out the nitrogen.

Nor can the body store surplus protein. In the short term, protein is converted into glucose in the liver or directly combines with oxygen to provide heat and energy. Any protein that is not used in this way is converted to fat and stored. Therefore, in terms of food costs and of the risk to health, eating too much protein is an expensive way of obtaining energy. In addi-

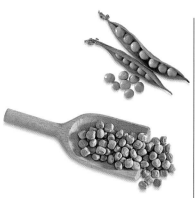

PODS AND LEGUMES
Legumes are the seeds of pod-bearing plants. But, whether a pea or a bean is fresh, frozen, or dried, it contains the same amount of protein.

tion, animal protein, such as fatty meat and full-fat dairy products, is almost always associated with high levels of saturated fat. So the more animal protein in your diet, the more saturated fat you consume. In the long term, diets high in saturated fat have been linked to heart disease and strokes.

High-protein (amino acid) supplements are often taken by athletes in the mistaken belief that this is the quickest way to make them stronger and more muscular. But consuming large amounts of protein does not help build more muscle: only exercise can build more muscle cells. Instead, athletes and other individuals interested in body building in particular should eat more carbohydrate-rich foods, such as pasta, to provide them with the energy to carry out their intensive exercise programs.

Studies have shown that eating too many protein-rich foods or taking purified amino acid supplements encourages the body to lose calcium in urine. Excess calcium loss causes osteoporosis (thinning of the bones), a serious condition that is on the rise among postmenopausal women (see page 69). Sufferers should avoid high-protein foods, and make sure that they have sufficient intakes of calcium and vitamin D.

Pathway to health

Gout is a very painful disease caused by excess uric acid in the blood. Uric acid crystals then form in joints, particularly the big toe, and the joints become inflamed, swollen, and very tender. The sufferer often experiences extreme pain and may be unable to put any pressure on the affected area. Usually the first attack of gout affects only a single joint. If there are subsequent attacks, more joints may become affected.

Uric acid is made from the breakdown of nucleic acids. A number of protein foods contain byproducts of this breakdown called purines, and some doctors recommend that gout sufferers avoid these foods. Included in this group are liver, kidneys, and other organ meats, sardines, anchovies, and dried legumes. Red wine, beer, and other alcoholic beverages may also be culprits. Sufferers of gout should drink plenty of nonalcoholic fluids to prevent buildup of uric acid, and shed excess pounds, which can aggravate the condition.

MEATLESS PROTEIN BOOSTS

If you want to restrict your meat intake but still retain sufficient protein in your diet, try the combinations below. Also, keep in mind that a small quantity of a complete protein food such as meat or cheese added to a less complete one—beans, peas, rice—will enhance the quality of the incomplete food. You get plenty of protein while reducing the cost and saturated fat content of the dish.

▶ *Beans and grains—try tofu, lentils, or beans served with rice, and falafel (deep-fried chickpea balls) with pita bread. Because soybeans have a 41 to 50 percent protein content, soy products such as soy milk, soy yogurt, and soybean curd (tofu) are popular with people who want to curtail their meat consumption.*

▶ *Seeds or nuts and beans—the Middle Eastern dish hummus (chickpea and sesame seed spread) and Chinese bean curd with sesame seeds are two popular combinations.*

▶ *Peanuts and grains—peanuts, which fall into the category of legumes, provide almost as much protein as beef when combined with grains. Spread peanut butter on whole-grain toast for a nourishing snack.*

MEXICAN DELIGHT
This hearty meal, which combines taco shells and beans, provides good-quality protein. Add some low-fat yogurt and plenty of vegetables for a well-balanced meal.

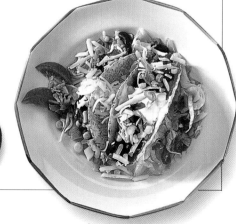

The Vegetarian Body Builder

The major source of protein for most people is meat and dairy products, so vegetarians may well ask, "How will I get enough protein?" For vegetarians who work out with weights, this question seems all the more pressing. After all, many of us assume that bodybuilders are supposed to follow a protein-rich diet.

Paul is 29 and single. Since his college days he has been a vegetarian. Last year Paul noticed that he was gaining weight. His friend Simon suggested he join a gym, and since then Paul has been lifting weights three times a week.

Although Paul made progress in the first few months, gradually his weight loss slowed and he had less stamina. Simon suggested that the lack of protein in Paul's vegetarian diet was causing the problem.

Because Paul does not eat meat, he decided to try amino acid supplements, which are available at drugstores and health food stores. After a few weeks he started to develop migraines, lost his appetite, and had less energy. Now he is worried that something is wrong.

WHAT SHOULD PAUL DO?

Paul should make an appointment with his doctor to establish the cause of his symptoms. His doctor can also refer him to a dietitian. Analyzing his diet will help Paul to find out whether he really does need to boost his protein intake with amino acid supplements.

Paul needs to consider whether weight training alone will help him to overcome his problem of excess weight. With his trainer Paul could devise a new program that will help him to further his gains in strength and stamina. He needs to investigate whether an aerobic exercise such as swimming or cycling will help to reduce his weight and keep it stable more effectively than just weight training.

Action Plan

HEALTH
Consult a doctor to find out what is the cause of the migraines, appetite loss, and lack of energy.

DIET
Consult a dietitian to find out whether his diet contains sufficient protein. (The dietitian will teach Paul how to choose and combine vegetarian foods for a nutritionally well-balanced diet.)

FITNESS
Find out about other forms of exercise that will help reduce weight and increase stamina. See whether the sports center has aerobics classes.

DIET
Lacking protein-rich meat in their diets, vegetarians need to make sure they are consuming the right combinations of plant proteins.

HEALTH
Supplements can cause problems such as migraine headaches in susceptible people. It is wise to check with a doctor or dietitian before taking them.

HOW THINGS TURN OUT FOR PAUL

Paul's doctor explained that the supplements contributed to his symptoms and would not aid muscle growth. His trainer suggested that on the days he did not work out, Paul could swim or cycle for at least half an hour to help him lose weight. Paul visited a dietitian, who confirmed that his diet, which includes plenty of beans and wheat, is providing him with sufficient protein calories. After a few days without the supplements, Paul found the migraines had disappeared.

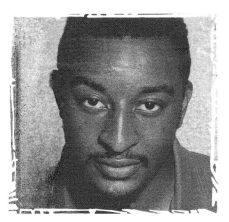

FITNESS
Following a single exercise program may not be the best way of increasing stamina.

VEGETARIANISM

No longer viewed as just for eccentrics, a meatless diet is growing ever more popular, particularly with the young, as researchers discover the health benefits of meat-free eating.

WHAT IS A VEGETARIAN?

By definition, vegetarianism prohibits the consumption of meat or fish, but some diets are more restrictive than others.

▶ *Demi- or semi-vegetarians eat fish and sometimes chicken but not red meat.*

▶ *Ovo-lacto-vegetarians include milk and eggs in their diet but not meat or fish.*

▶ *Lacto-vegetarians consume milk and yogurt, as well as cheese made with vegetarian rennet, but no meat, fish, or eggs.*

▶ *Vegans do not eat any animal products at all, banning meat, fish, milk, and eggs from their diets.*

▶ *Fruitarians exclude legumes and cereals from the diet, as well as all foods of animal origin. Fruitarians eat only fruit, honey, nuts, and nut oils.*

▶ *Macrobiotic followers have a regimen that becomes progressively more restrictive through 10 different levels. At first, animal foods are excluded, then fruit and vegetables as well. At the final, "purist" level only brown rice is eaten.*

In the United States about 12.4 million people (about 5 percent of the population) call themselves vegetarians. In the United Kingdom the number of people making this claim is about 2.5 million (about 4.3 percent of the population), and in Germany about 2.9 million people (4.5 percent of the population) say they do not eat meat.

THE HEALTH BENEFITS

On the whole, vegetarians tend to follow current healthy eating guidelines. Because they do not eat meat, a prime source of saturated fat, vegetarians take in less total fat and more fiber, in the form of fruits, vegetables, and whole-grain cereals. These foods are also good sources of beta carotene, vitamin C, and vitamin E, which are antioxidant nutrients and may protect the body from disease (see page 94).

The Oxford Vegetarian Study, a long-term project set up in 1980 by researchers at Oxford University, has collected information on the health and mortality of more than 6,000 vegetarian subjects and a control group of more than 5,000 meat-eating individuals. Allowing for smoking habits, body mass index, and social class—all factors that influence mortality rates—the study has revealed significant differences between the two groups. For example, in contrast to meat eaters, vegetarians have a 39 percent lower risk of dying from cancer.

The study's data also found that the risk of heart disease was 24 percent lower in vegetarians and 57 percent lower in vegans than in regular meat eaters. And when they compared blood cholesterol concentrations, researchers found that vegetarians, particularly vegans, had lower levels of low-density

SUGGESTED FOOD SERVINGS FOR VEGETARIANS

The types of foods eaten by vegetarians can be organized into five groups as in the Food Guide Pyramid on page 18. For a well-balanced diet, choose foods from the different groups in the daily proportions recommended here. This eating plan may be adapted for vegans, who should select greater quantities of foods from the protein (peas, beans) and carbohydrate (bread) groups.

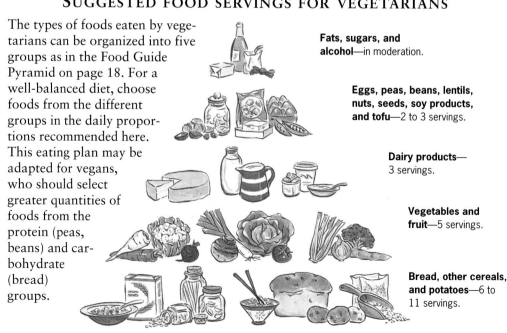

Fats, sugars, and alcohol—in moderation.

Eggs, peas, beans, lentils, nuts, seeds, soy products, and tofu—2 to 3 servings.

Dairy products— 3 servings.

Vegetables and fruit—5 servings.

Bread, other cereals, and potatoes—6 to 11 servings.

lipoproteins (LDL's)—the "bad" blood cholesterol, which is a primary risk factor in heart disease (see page 56).

Another major study of 1,900 vegetarians was conducted at the German Cancer Research Center in 1978. The researchers found that the rate of cardiovascular disease was 61 percent lower in male vegetarians and 44 percent lower in female vegetarians than in the general population. The men in the study had a greatly reduced cancer death rate—about half the national average—and the women's cancer mortality rate was reduced by one quarter.

A vegetarian diet may also confer some protection against colon cancer, and much research is being undertaken to determine why. A professor at the Harvard Medical School, Walter C. Willet, studied more than 88,000 women aged 34 to 59 years. The results showed that daily consumption of red meat more than doubled the risk of developing colon cancer, compared with eating this food less than once a week. But meat eaters usually eat fewer vegetables than vegetarians. And it may be the lack of vegetables eaten rather than an excess of meat that was of significance in the study. Vegetables are a rich source of the antioxidants that may help to prevent cancer. The high-fiber and complex-carbohydrate intake among vegetarians is considered to be another factor in lowering their risk of colon cancer.

Some researchers claim that premature death by cancer and heart disease is only part of the story for meat eaters. Eating a high-protein diet may have other harmful consequences. For example, calcium loss and increased uric acid as a result of eating too much protein may be a cause of kidney stone formation and kidney failure.

A vegetarian diet may help to relieve the symptoms of rheumatoid arthritis, according to Dr. Jens Kjeldsen-Kragh of the Institute of Immunology and Rheumatology at the National Hospital, Oslo, Norway. He found in 1991 that patients on an established vegetarian diet experienced less pain and stiffness and fewer swollen joints. However, sufferers of other types of arthritis, such as ankylosing spondylitis, appear to benefit from a high-meat, low complex-carbohydrate diet.

Citing these studies and many others, researchers now believe that vegetarianism

SOURCES OF PROTEIN IN A DAILY MENU

Many foods beside meat provide protein. The meals below contain a range of simple, nourishing foods that supply an adequate intake of protein.

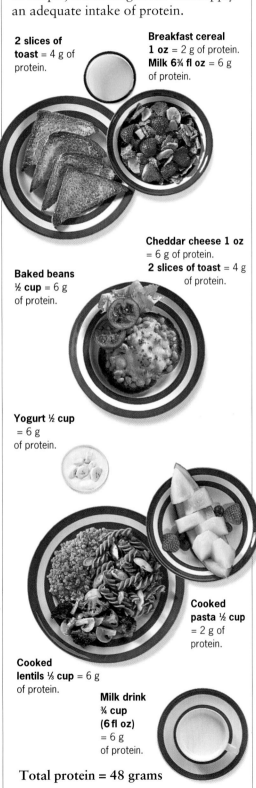

2 slices of toast = 4 g of protein.

Breakfast cereal 1 oz = 2 g of protein.
Milk 6¾ fl oz = 6 g of protein.

Cheddar cheese 1 oz = 6 g of protein.
2 slices of toast = 4 g of protein.

Baked beans ½ cup = 6 g of protein.

Yogurt ½ cup = 6 g of protein.

Cooked pasta ½ cup = 2 g of protein.

Cooked lentils ⅓ cup = 6 g of protein.

Milk drink ¾ cup (6 fl oz) = 6 g of protein.

Total protein = 48 grams

Vegetarian cheese

Rennet, which is used in cheese making, traditionally comes from the stomach lining of cows. Strict vegetarians often refuse to eat ordinary cheese because it contains this animal product. Luckily, cheeses are now available made with vegetarian rennet, which is genetically engineered from microorganisms and therefore does not require the rennet from animal sources.

Textured vegetable protein

An inexpensive alternative to meat, textured vegetable protein (TVP) is made from soybeans. First the oil is extracted and refined to make vegetable oil. Then the residue is processed to extract the protein, which is formed into a white spongy product that is available in an assortment of shapes and sizes. TVP is usually fortified with B vitamins and iron.

USING TEXTURED VEGETABLE PROTEIN
After soaking, TVP can be cooked in a variety of ways—try combining it with nuts and dried beans in casseroles and roasts or use it to make vegetarian burgers.

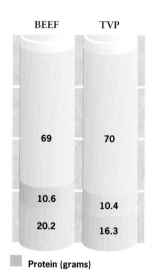

BEEF	TVP
69	70
10.6	10.4
20.2	16.3

■ Protein (grams)
■ Fat (grams)
■ Moisture (grams)
■ Carbohydrate (grams)

NUTRITIONAL VALUES
The bar chart above compares the nutritional content of beef and TVP.

may promote longevity. But their diet may not be the only reason why vegetarians are healthier than meat eaters. Vegetarians tend also to live "healthier" lives—smoking and drinking alcohol less and exercising more.

Meeting your needs

With all these health benefits, it is little wonder that vegetarianism is on the rise. But you still need a balanced diet to remain healthy. It is not enough just to stop eating animal flesh and consume a few high-protein foods, such as cheese, instead. Cheese, like meat, contains a lot of fat, particularly saturated fat, which is linked to heart disease and cancer. Choose low-fat dairy products such as skim milk or nonfat yogurt, and make sure that your diet includes foods from all the main vegetarian food groups: fruit and vegetables; nuts, seeds, dried peas, beans and lentils, and soy products; grains and cereals; and dairy products. With a little planning, you can make nourishing meals using a variety of fresh foods.

Missing nutrients?

Some people believe that a vegetarian diet does not offer an adequate supply of vitamins and minerals. But by eating a variety of foods vegetarians should get all the nutrients they need. They do have an increased risk of iron and zinc deficiency, however, especially if they eat large amounts of unleavened bread, for example, pita bread. These foods contain phytic acid, which inhibits mineral absorption.

Vegans also may not get enough vitamin B_{12}. A prolonged deficiency of this vitamin can seriously impair the body's central nervous system, causing numbness in the limbs. In addition, there may be neurological signs such as loss of memory. Those at risk should seek out foods that are fortified with vitamin B_{12} during processing. Some possibilities are vegetarian burgers, breakfast cereals, yeast extract, and soy milk.

A good supply of vitamin D is essential for the healthy maintenance of bones. Any person, vegetarian or otherwise, who receives a sufficient amount of sunlight can synthesize adequate amounts of vitamin D. Just 15 minutes of sunlight each day is enough for most people. When sunlight isn't available, dairy products and margarines fortified with vitamin D can help. Some vegetarians, especially those on a macrobiotic diet, may require supplements as well. If you are in doubt, consult your doctor.

A VEGETARIAN IN THE FAMILY

Preparing and cooking meals for a vegetarian is easy, even if everybody else eats meat. And meat eaters in the family may be persuaded to become "part-time vegetarians" if you have one or two meat-free days a week.

While many meals can be prepared without using any animal products, it is also possible to organize your meals so that you cater to both meat eaters and vegetarians with essentially the same dish. Instead of cooking two different meals, prepare a meat-free sauce, rice dish, or casserole, then divide it. Add beans and vegetables to one portion and meat or fish to the other.

When making meat-free stews or soups, cook twice as much as you need and freeze the remainder in meal-size portions. These can be defrosted when you need a substitute for a meat dish for one member of the family. Leftover vegetable or textured vegetable protein mixtures can be used as alternative fillings for pies, bell peppers, or crepes traditionally filled with meat.

SATISFYING DIFFERENT TASTES
Baked potatoes make a hearty meal and can be dressed with a variety of simple, nutritious toppings suitable for both vegetarians and meat eaters.

For a meat eater, just add ground lean beef or chopped poultry to the vegetarian sauce.

For a vegetarian, try beans lightly cooked with tomatoes, herbs, and bell peppers.

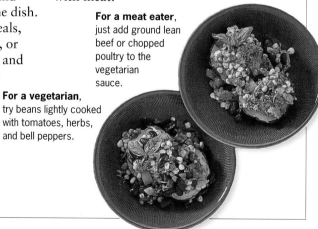

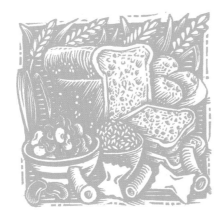

CHAPTER 3

THE OPTIMUM BODY FUEL— CARBOHYDRATES

Worldwide, carbohydrates make up about 75 percent of total calorie intake, but in the developed world they comprise only 45 percent, with almost half coming from sugar. One reason for these numbers is that many people have long perceived starchy foods such as bread, potatoes, and pasta as fattening. We now know that the complex carbohydrates of grains and vegetables provide the body with a steady flow of the fuel it needs to function smoothly, and the unprocessed forms provide needed fiber as well.

THE ENERGY FOODS

Although starchy and sweet foods look and taste different, all are made primarily of the same building block—sugar—the body's best source of energy.

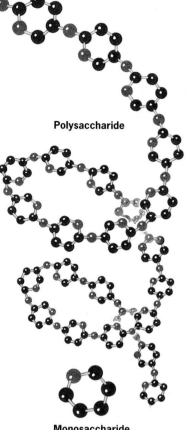

Polysaccharide

Monosaccharide

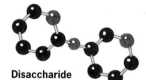

Disaccharide

SUGAR UNITS
All carbohydrates are made up of molecules called saccharides. Simple sugars, such as glucose and fructose, consist of single ringlike units (monosaccharides). Table sugar (sucrose) is a disaccharide. It is made up of two saccharides, glucose and fructose, connected by an oxygen molecule. Complex carbohydrates, or polysaccharides, are long, spiraling chains of many connecting monosaccharides.

Whenever you lift a weight, take a walk, or run for a bus, your body burns glucose, its primary source of energy. Glucose is found in carbohydrates, a group of foods with identical chemical components that is divided into two categories: simple sugars and complex carbohydrates. The simplest of sugars, monosaccharides, consist of single molecules and include glucose, fructose, and galactose. Disaccharides, which form when two molecules join up, include sucrose (table sugar), lactose (milk sugar), and maltose (malt sugar). Complex carbohydrates, also known as starches, are made up of at least 10 saccharides and are found in plant foods like wheat, rice, potatoes, corn, beans, and yams. Unrefined carbohydrates, including whole-grain cereals, and breads and brown rice, are highly nutritious. However, when refined, as white sugar and white flour, carbohydrates lose much of their nutritional value.

Glucose occurs naturally only in fruits and honey and is the only carbohydrate used by the body to generate energy. Most carbohydrates are broken down into glucose when they are digested; the rest are

IS SUGAR BAD FOR HEALTH?

Sugar has been accused of contributing to many diseases and disorders, including diabetes, heart disease, hypertension, and hyperactivity in children. But research studies have not provided evidence that sugar actually causes any of these conditions. What most nutritionists will confirm, however, is that the frequent consumption of sugar accelerates tooth decay.

Everybody has bacteria in the mouth that can lead to plaque (a film of mucus) on teeth. Sugar or starch that remains in the mouth becomes easily accessible food for the bacteria, which produce an acid that damages tooth enamel and causes cavities. Tooth decay is most strongly linked to the frequency of sugar consumption and the propensity for the sweet foods to cling to the teeth. Candies and chewing gum, therefore, are more cariogenic than cakes.

It is better if sweet foods or sugary drinks are consumed with meals rather than between meals.

The role of sugar in obesity is more complex, since it is the total number of calories consumed that is important, rather than the calorie source. However, many sugary foods, such as ice cream, cookies, cakes, and chocolates, are high in fat; people who eat and drink large amounts of them may find that cutting down on these foods aids weight loss.

DENTAL FLOSSING
Acid forms on teeth only if plaque is present. It is important to clean and floss your teeth regularly to remove plaque.

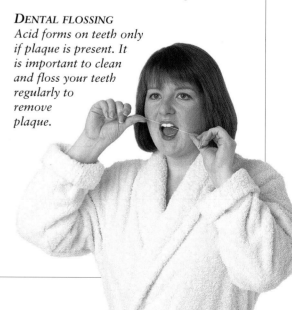

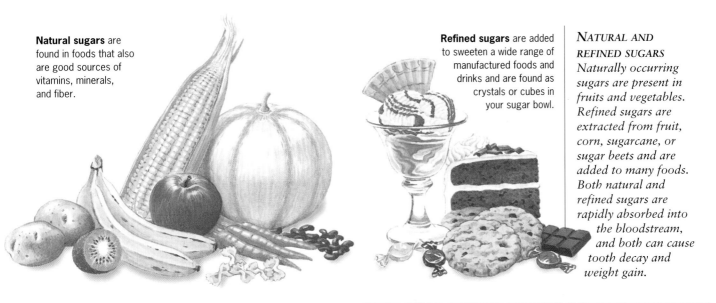

Natural sugars are found in foods that also are good sources of vitamins, minerals, and fiber.

Refined sugars are added to sweeten a wide range of manufactured foods and drinks and are found as crystals or cubes in your sugar bowl.

NATURAL AND REFINED SUGARS Naturally occurring sugars are present in fruits and vegetables. Refined sugars are extracted from fruit, corn, sugarcane, or sugar beets and are added to many foods. Both natural and refined sugars are rapidly absorbed into the bloodstream, and both can cause tooth decay and weight gain.

THE CARBOHYDRATE CONTENT OF FOOD

Many foods contain both simple sugars and complex carbohydrates, and the relative proportions of these are shown in the table below. Foods at the top of the table are high in sugars, while those at the bottom are high in starches. Think of the table as a traffic light, with "red" at the top, "yellow" in the center, and "green" (for go) foods at the bottom. Ideally, you should eat no more than 2 ounces of added refined sugar a day, preferably in high-fiber desserts, cakes, and cookies, such as oatmeal cookies and banana bread.

FOOD	COMPLEX CARBOHYDRATES grams per portion	SUGARS grams per portion	COMMENTS
"RED" FOODS			
Hard candy, 1 oz	0.0	18.9	Almost pure sugar.
Peaches, canned in syrup, ½ cup	1.5	24.0	At least half the sugar is added.
Sweetened puffed wheat cereal, 1 oz	8.9	16.3	High in added sugar and low in fiber.
Sponge cake, 1 slice	10.2	21.1	Most cakes and cookies are high in added sugar.
"YELLOW" FOODS			
Fruit yogurt, 8 oz	8.5	34.7	Unflavored yogurt with fresh fruit is preferable.
Banana, 1 medium	8.9	17.8	Sugars in fruit and vegetables are encouraged.
Baked beans, 1 cup	37.7	14.4	Added sugar makes beans palatable, particularly for children.
"GREEN" FOODS			
Sweet corn, cooked, ½ cup	18.5	2.1	Excellent sources of complex carbohydrates, these foods also provide other important nutrients, including protein. Bread and brown rice contain niacin, riboflavin, other B vitamins, and usually some iron; potatoes and corn have fair amounts of potassium and Vitamin C. All unrefined, complex-carbohydrate foods are good sources of dietary fiber.
Baked potato with skin, 1 medium	51.0	3.2	
Pasta, white, cooked, 1 cup	30.2	1.8	
Rice, brown, cooked, 1 cup	44.2	0.6	
Rice, white, cooked, 1 cup	45.0	0.3	
Bread, whole-wheat, 1 slice	10.3	1.0	
Bread, white, 1 slice	11.4	1.0	

Sweeteners

Manufacturers add sugar as a sweetener to many different processed foods. But it is not always easy to know that they have done so, since sugar is listed on the label under many different names. For example, corn syrup, dextrose, maltose, maltodextrin, glucose syrup, invert sugars, and levulose are all forms of sugar.

SPICED DELIGHT
Use flavorings such as cinnamon, allspice, cardamom, cloves, ginger, and nutmeg when you prepare foods and reduce your sugar intake without reducing flavor.

changed to glucose in the liver. If the body does not need carbohydrates for energy immediately, the muscles and liver store them as glycogen, which then provides energy when the body demands it. Any surplus glucose is eventually converted to fat and stored in the body.

Extra goodness

Unrefined complex-carbohydrate foods are particularly good for you because they are usually full of fiber. Dietary fiber plays an important role in bowel function (see page 46). Research suggests that insoluble fiber may help to prevent some types of cancer and soluble fiber may help to lower the blood cholesterol level. In addition, complex-carbohydrate foods such as bread, rice, dried beans, and root vegetables provide not only starch and fiber but also essential vitamins and minerals.

A CHANGE FOR THE WORSE

In affluent societies, the most dramatic dietary change in the past 100 years has been the switch from foods high in complex carbohydrates to foods that are high in fat and sugar. These high-fat, simple-carbohydrate diets are generally low in fiber. The combination of these factors is thought to contribute to many contemporary health concerns—particularly tooth decay, heart disease, cancer, and bowel disorders—that have arisen over the same period. Most health experts recommend returning to a diet more like that of agricultural societies —with more complex-carbohydrate foods and less sugar and fat.

Added sugar: sweet poison

Manufacturers often add refined sugar to food because it has important preservative properties; it also adds bulk and viscosity, and—in cookies, cakes, and quick breads—tenderness. Fruit yogurts, for example, may contain the equivalent of 5 teaspoons of sugar. Sweetening plain yogurt with your own fresh fruit, such as blueberries, apricots, or strawberries, presents a much healthier alternative.

Unlike foods rich in complex carbohydrates, those high in refined sugars are usually poor sources of other nutrients; for this reason, they are often called "empty calories." Foods such as cakes, cookies, doughnuts, sweets, and chocolate are high in refined sugar, with few, if any, compensating nutrients or dietary fiber.

Certain foods, such as baked beans and some high-fiber breakfast cereals, contain added simple sugars to make them tastier. However, since these foods are a good source of other important nutrients and the amount of sugar is not excessive, they can still be a valuable part of a healthy diet. So, too, can foods that contain natural sugars—fruit and milk, for example (especially reduced-fat milk). Both offer vitamins, minerals and, in the case of milk, protein. Fruit, of course, also has fiber.

MORE THAN JUST DAILY BREAD

There are a number of ways that you can add more complex-carbohydrate foods to your diet while cutting down on fatty and sugary foods. All types of bread are good for you, especially whole-grain varieties.

SATISFYING YOUR SWEET TOOTH

From birth, babies seem to prefer sweet to sour tastes. Most adults and almost all children enjoy sweet-tasting foods. But cutting back on sugar does not mean denying yourself sweet foods or desserts. Fruits contain natural sugars, so by using unsweetened fruit juice, fresh fruit, and unsweetened canned fruit to replace refined sugars in recipes, you satisfy your sweet tooth without harming your health. The benefits are obvious—less tooth decay and more vitamins and fiber.

Here are some suggestions:

► *If fresh fruit is unavailable, eat fruits canned in water or juice rather than syrup.*

► *Substitute fresh fruit purees for sugar in recipes, if possible.*

► *Add fresh fruit to plain yogurt.*

► *Sprinkle sweet spices on foods, for example, cinnamon on baked apples.*

► *Add dried fruit, such as raisins and figs, to breakfast cereals.*

► *Use no-sugar-added jams when possible.*

Although mills often fortify refined flour with vitamins and minerals—usually niacin, thiamin, riboflavin, and iron—to replace nutrients lost during refining, they never quite succeed in duplicating what nature created. Stone-ground whole-wheat flour, for example, retains as much as 90 percent of its original nutrients plus the fiber.

If you start the day with cereal, you will have a steady stream of energy during the morning. Oatmeal and other whole-grain breakfast cereals are full of nutrients as well as complex carbohydrates. And by eating them with low-fat or nonfat milk, you will avoid taking in unneeded fat. Then, during the day, choose snacks that are rich in complex carbohydrates and low in fat. Air-popped popcorn, toasted pumpkin seeds, breadsticks, and soft unsalted pretzels are both satisfying and good for you.

Cooked beans provide both starch and fiber. When making meat dishes, replace one-third of the meat with cooked beans. Also add beans to salads, soups, and stews, and purée them to make spreads and dips.

For desserts that have more than empty calories, incorporate fruit and/or milk. Try frozen low-fat yogurt, and sweeten rice pudding with fresh or dried fruit.

LOSING WEIGHT

Foods high in complex carbohydrates can be a boon to people who want to lose weight, because most of these foods are filling, chewy, and full of fiber and other nutrients. However, portion sizes are important. A 3-ounce serving of pasta with

---

DOES YOUR CARBOHYDRATE INTAKE MEASURE UP?

The current recommendations for healthy eating suggest that you should obtain about 55 percent of your energy needs (calories) from carbohydrates. Most nutritionists agree that refined sugars should consist of about 10 percent of your calorie intake and complex carbohydrates about 45 percent.

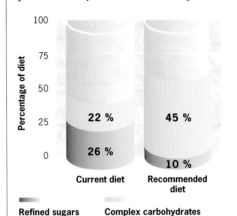

Percentage of diet

	Current diet	Recommended diet
	22 %	45 %
	26 %	10 %

▬ Refined sugars   ▬ Complex carbohydrates

INCREASING YOUR INTAKE
This chart shows how many people's diets compare with the recommended diet in terms of carbohydrate intake.

Moral crusade
During the 19th century, a crusade against refined wheat flour was led by the Reverend Sylvester Graham (1794–1851). A Presbyterian minister from Philadelphia, Graham fiercely condemned white bread, claiming it was contributing to the downfall of society.

Graham described the refining process as putting "asunder what God had joined together." He encouraged people to eat more whole-grain bread and wrote a long treatise on its importance for the moral, spiritual, and physical welfare of mankind. Subsequently, whole-wheat flour was named after him, and all Americans are familiar with the "graham cracker"—a healthful, whole-wheat cookie.

---

a simple tomato sauce has about 450 calories; a 5-ounce serving (typical of many restaurant dishes) has about 750, or more than a third of many people's daily caloric total. Nutritionists now know that it is the total calorie content of the diet, along with

---

PUTTING HEALTH ON YOUR PLATE

Most people should eat plenty of complex-carbohydrate foods. One of the easiest ways to do this is to rethink the proportions of food you put on your plate. Rice, pasta, bread, and potatoes should fill two-fifths of the plate; vegetables or salad should make up at least another two-fifths; and meat, fish, cheese, or eggs, the remainder.

IN THE RIGHT PROPORTION
When serving meals, try to make sure the portions of complex-carbohydrate foods, vegetables or salad, and protein foods on each plate match the amounts shown here.

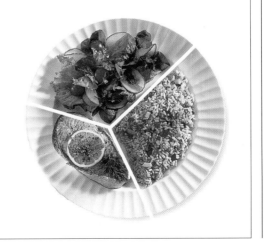

The potato: the dieter's friend

Ounce for ounce, gram for gram, fatty foods are more than twice as high in calories as complex carbohydrates. But while starchy foods such as pasta and potatoes are naturally low in calories, adding butter or an oily dressing negates this benefit.

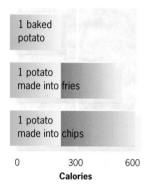

1 baked potato		
1 potato made into fries		
1 potato made into chips		

0　　　300　　　600
Calories

ACCUMULATING CALORIES
An average baked potato provides about 200 calories. Once peeled and fried, the same potato offers about 500 calories; if made into potato chips, the potato would then be valued at 600 calories.

the amount of exercise, that determines whether a person is likely to lose, maintain, or gain weight, and that fat is often the culprit in overweight or obesity. Reducing your fat intake is one of the best ways to reduce your total calorie intake, because 1 gram of fat has 9 calories whereas 1 gram of carbohydrate or protein has 4 calories.

Proteins versus carbohydrates

Dieters were once encouraged to make their meals high in protein rather than carbohydrates, and many people still believe that such a regimen will be successful. However, high-protein foods like meat and cheese are often high in fat and therefore, calories. Diets high in protein and low in carbohydrates are also likely to be low in fiber, thus allowing waste products to build up.

Most experts argue that weight loss is most easily achieved by cutting down on the intake of fat without altering the intake of carbohydrates. For a diet to be success-

Pathway to health

If you are very concerned about being overweight, talk to your doctor and ask him or her to refer you to a dietitian. The dietitian will recommend a weight-loss diet that best suits your needs and lifestyle and will also monitor your progress.

ful, however, dieters must be careful to cook or dress the carbohydrate foods with minimal quantities of oil or butter.

There is actually a danger to a diet that is too low in carbohydrates. Their limited availability forces the body to make glucose out of protein and fat, and high levels of waste products called ketones build up. The ketones can cause nausea, fatigue, and headache. Also, excess protein puts a strain on the kidneys, which have to filter out the extra waste matter (see page 33).

Large quantities of low-fat, high-bulk foods are more likely to help you lose weight. In one experiment, a group of young Irishmen were put on a diet that involved eating about 2 pounds (just under 1 kilogram) of potatoes per day for three months. Provided that they ate the potatoes, they could eat as much other food as they wanted. However, after three months most of the men had lost weight. They found that by filling themselves up with the potatoes, they automatically reduced their total intake of higher-calorie foods.

It is not easy to lose weight. A strict dietary regimen for a few weeks often results in the loss of a few pounds, but the pounds soon creep back when people return to their previous dietary habits. Changing your diet over the long term to one that is high in complex carbohydrates and lower in foods with a high-fat content is a more successful way to maintain weight loss.

"HEAVEN'S GIFT"

Honey is a smooth, sticky sweetener that the Roman poet Virgil called "heaven's gift." It has been used by humans for thousands of years to sweeten cakes and pastries, and to flavor candies, glazes, butters, and liqueurs.

The simple sugars glucose and fructose, which give honey its sweetness, taste even sweeter than table sugar (sucrose, also a simple sugar). For this reason, less of it than of other sugars is needed to sweeten food. Also, because honey has a high-water content, it contains fewer calories than an equal weight of sugar. There are 385 calories in 3½ ounces of table sugar, but only 304 calories in 3½ ounces of honey. However, honey is still a sugar, so its use should be limited.

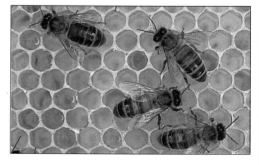

HONEYCOMB
Worker honeybees fill the honeycomb, a waxy cylindrical network, with nectar from flowers. The chambers are capped with wax, and the honey is left to ripen for a few weeks.

CALORIE COMPARISON

The two diets below have identical calorie counts and sufficient protein, vitamins, and minerals. But the diet that is higher in whole grains has more bulk, and so is more satisfying and nutritionally better. Note that light meals are served for dinner.

DIET ONE
A diet high in complex carbohydrates.

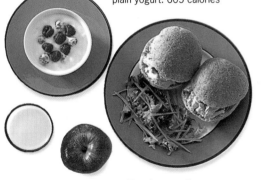

Breakfast
1 oz whole-wheat cereal
with low-fat milk and 1 sliced small banana;
1 slice whole-wheat bread or toast with 1 tsp butter
or margarine; coffee with low-fat milk. 355 calories

Midmorning
Coffee with 2 tbsp low-fat
milk. 15 calories

Lunch
2 whole-grain rolls with 1 tsp
mayonnaise, filled with 4 oz
tuna and plain yogurt,
and a small salad; 8 fl oz
low-fat milk, 1 apple, and 5 fl oz
plain yogurt. 605 calories

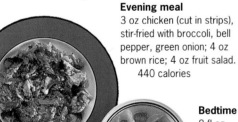

Evening meal
3 oz chicken (cut in strips),
stir-fried with broccoli, bell
pepper, green onion; 4 oz
brown rice; 4 oz fruit salad.
440 calories

Bedtime
8 fl oz
low-fat milk.
115 calories

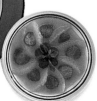

Total calories = 1,530

DIET TWO
A diet low in complex carbohydrates.

Breakfast
1 oz breakfast
cereal with low-fat milk;
1 slice white toast with 1 tsp butter or margarine;
4 fl oz fruit juice (orange); coffee with
low-fat milk. 350 calories

Midmorning
Coffee with 2 tbsp low-fat
milk. 15 calories

Lunch
1 white roll with 1 tsp
mayonnaise, filled with 1 oz
Cheddar cheese and salad;
8 fl oz low-fat milk, 1 banana,
and fruit-flavored yogurt.
595 calories

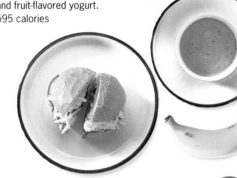

Evening meal
8 oz broiled rump
steak; 3½ oz green
salad with 1 tbsp
of vinaigrette
dressing; 8 fl oz
tomato juice.
455 calories

Bedtime
8 fl oz low-fat milk. 115 calories

Total calories = 1,530

Artificial sugars
If you want to reduce your intake of table sugar, you can add artificial sugars, such as aspartame and saccharin, to drinks and cold foods instead. They are also used by manufacturers to sweeten diet soft drinks and other "low-calorie" foods.

Saccharin has been available for 50 years and is generally considered to be safe. Although studies on laboratory rats have shown that large quantities can cause bladder cancer, there have been no reports of it causing cancer in humans.

Aspartame, also considered safe, is made up of two amino acids—aspartic acid and phenylalanine. Its amino acids are used by the body in the same way as other amino acids (see page 30).

Both saccharin and aspartame are 200 times sweeter than sugar but do not cause tooth decay. Still, some experts consider it unwise to consume large quantities of artificial sweeteners habitually, because the long-term effects of high intakes in humans are still unknown.

THE FIBER FACTOR

During the 1980's, fiber was hailed as a way to halt heart disease and colon cancer and to lower cholesterol. But in spite of this, many people have only slightly increased their fiber intake.

Oat bran
As a rich source of soluble fiber, oat bran is a valuable ally in the battle against excessive levels of harmful forms of cholesterol. In the 1980's medical reports trumpeting its particular benefits brought about a huge increase in its consumption. In fact, other foods that are high in soluble fiber—such as beans, apples, rolled oats, and potatoes—are just as valuable as oat bran for reducing blood cholesterol.

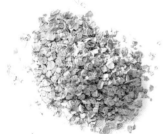

A VALUABLE INGREDIENT
On a cold day, a hot oat cereal makes a warming breakfast. Adding oats to dishes such as pancakes or apple crisp is another good way to boost the nutritional value with extra fiber.

Although the role that fiber plays in stimulating bowel function has been well known since ancient times, its significance for disease prevention is a more recent discovery. Two British doctors, Denis Burkitt and Hugh Trowell, are credited with bringing this to the attention of the public in the 1970's. Having worked extensively in East Africa, they put forward the theory that many diseases common in industrialized countries but rare in Africa might be partly caused by insufficient fiber in the Western diet. Further studies led to a consensus that people in the West could benefit from increasing the level of fiber content in their diets.

INSOLUBLE AND SOLUBLE FIBER
The word *fiber* refers to a range of plant materials—components of plant cell walls—that the human body cannot digest. Other terms that are used to describe dietary fiber are *roughage* and *nonstarch polysaccharides* (NSP). Most fiber compounds pass through the body unchanged until they reach the large intestine. Here, fibers act in different ways, depending on whether they are insoluble or soluble.

Insoluble fiber absorbs water, thus adding bulk to fecal matter in the bowel. This added bulk helps to stimulate the muscles of the lower digestive tract to move waste products more quickly. More important, insoluble fiber is fermented by the bacteria in the large bowel to produce fatty acids that nourish the intestinal wall.

Diets that are low in insoluble fiber are associated with the need to strain when passing a stool. Insufficient insoluble fiber is thought to contribute to such health problems as constipation, hemorrhoids, and diverticulosis (protruding pockets formed on the intestinal wall that are prone to infection). By speeding waste material

---

INSOLUBLE AND SOLUBLE FIBER IN FOODS

Brown rice, bran, whole-grain cereals and breads, and nuts are valuable sources of insoluble fiber. Soluble-fiber foods include oats, oat bran, peas, beans, root vegetables, and citrus fruits. Both types of fiber are found in apples, pears, barley, bananas, prunes, and the cabbage family.

HIGH-FIBER FOODS
The foods illustrated in the left circle provide insoluble fiber. The foods in the circle on the right are good sources of soluble fiber. In the middle are foods that provide both types of fiber.

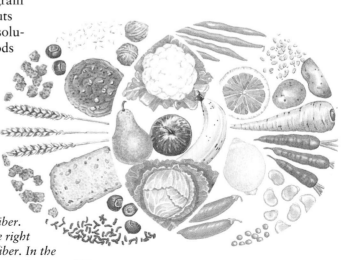

CLEARING OUT CHOLESTEROL

Soluble fiber binds cholesterol from the diet or from bile to prevent it being absorbed. The bound cholesterol is therefore excreted from the body in the feces. As the liver becomes partially depleted of cholesterol, it takes up cholesterol from the bloodstream, thus lowering the level of blood cholesterol.

FIBER AND FAT
Soluble fibers link with cholesterol and bile constituents to reduce cholesterol absorption.

Bile acids

Cholesterol

Soluble fibers
bind with cholesterol
and bile acids.

Large intestine

Slowly does it
Introduce high-fiber foods gradually into your diet to give your body time to adjust. You will also need to drink more, because fiber absorbs water. Because certain high-fiber foods—including dried peas, beans, and lentils—often lead to increased flatulence, you may want to begin by eating more cereals, grains, vegetables, and fruits and then add beans later.

through the body and therefore helping to prevent toxins from coming into prolonged contact with the intestinal wall, insoluble fiber may also protect against cancer of the lower bowel.

Soluble-fiber compounds, as the term suggests, break down somewhat in the digestive tract and form fatty acids, which are absorbed into the bloodstream. These fatty acids are thought to help reduce the total level of cholesterol in the blood and therefore lower the risk of heart and arterial disease. In one study of men with high cholesterol levels, adding ½ cup of cooked dried beans per day to their normal food intake reduced blood cholesterol levels by 13 percent in 21 days.

Soluble fiber is also thought to retard absorption of glucose into the bloodstream, helping to prevent diabetes mellitus and low blood sugar levels (hypoglycemia).

HIGH FIBER AND WEIGHT LOSS

Foods that are high in fiber are generally filling and low in fat and so can help to reduce total calorie intake. The chewiness of high-fiber foods prolongs eating time. Eating more slowly in turn gives your body time to tell your brain that your stomach is full. If you eat higher-fiber foods, you can have larger portions for the same calorie intake as from refined foods. For example, four 1-ounce cookies provide the same calorie value (140 calories) as two 1-ounce slices of whole-grain bread, or a 4-ounce baked potato eaten with its skin.

Since there are several ways of measuring the fiber content of foods, official recommendations about how much fiber to eat tend to vary from country to country. Generally speaking, 30 grams of fiber is a reasonable goal—a third as much again as adults in the developed world typically eat.

INCREASING THE FIBER IN YOUR DIET

Nutritionists recommend that everybody should eat 30 grams of fiber a day to help digestion, lower cholesterol, and prevent cancer of the bowel. Because people tend to eat too many refined foods, they miss out on the fiber they would get from unrefined products. An easy way to increase your intake of fiber is to include a variety of the foods listed at right in your daily diet. The food pyramid on page 18 will show you how to achieve the right balance.

CEREALS AND GRAINS
*All-bran breakfast cereal
(1 oz) = 8.5 g fiber
Whole-wheat spaghetti, cooked
(1 cup) = 4.5 g fiber
Whole-wheat bread
(2 slices) = 5.7 g fiber*

VEGETABLES AND FRUIT
*Dried apricots (½ cup) =
5.0 g fiber
Baked potato with skin (1 medium) =
5.0 g fiber
Apple with skin (1 medium) =
3.0 g fiber
Carrots, boiled (½ cup) = 2.9 g fiber
Green beans, boiled (½ cup) = 1.1 g fiber
Raspberries, raw (½ cup) = 2.8 g fiber*

PEAS, BEANS, AND LENTILS
*Red kidney beans or butter beans
(½ cup) = 4.3 g fiber
Lima beans, boiled
(½ cup) = 6.2 g fiber
Lentils, cooked
(½ cup) = 4.9 g fiber*

Eat apples with
their skins for
added fiber.

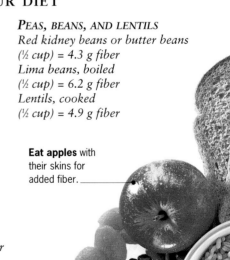

SUSTAINING ENERGY

Throughout the day, your energy level rises and falls as the sugars from carbohydrates you eat enter your bloodstream and are used to provide energy.

Glucose, or blood sugar, is the body's major source of energy; it's also the only form of energy that the brain can use effectively. During digestion and metabolism, the liver converts all of the carbohydrates and about half of the protein from a meal into glucose, which is then released into the bloodstream. In response to rising glucose levels, the pancreas secretes extra insulin, the hormone that enables cells to convert sugar into energy.

BLOOD-SUGAR LEVELS
Low blood sugar, or hypoglycemia, occurs when the amount of insulin exceeds what is needed to metabolize available glucose. This can happen when a person with diabetes takes too much insulin, and also when the body secretes more insulin than it needs, thus causing a drop in blood-glucose levels This last is called reactive hypoglycemia, and it is an unusual condition. Symptoms include dizziness, headache, trembling, palpitations, irritability, intense hunger, and mood swings. (A diabetic who takes an overdose of insulin may have similar but more pronounced symptoms.)

Reactive glycemia is rare, but some people experience mild symptoms of it due to stress, missed meals, or a low-calorie diet of mostly carbohydrates. For example, when a person has just juice and a sweet roll for breakfast, the pancreas will secrete a fair amount of insulin to process the meal, but as it contains no protein and little fat, which are metabolized more slowly than carbohydrates, the body will send out hunger signals within two or three hours. A sweet snack at this point will yield a quick burst of energy, but this, too, will dissipate quickly.

Such a cycle can be avoided by having regular meals that include protein, fat, and high-fiber carbohydrates, such as fresh fruit, vegetables, or whole-grain crackers or bread. Soluble fiber, especially, helps to ensure that glucose is absorbed into the bloodstream at a steady rate (see page 47). For diabetics, an insulin reaction can be alleviated by taking a little sugar, honey, a hard candy, juice, or a sugary soft drink.

EATING TO BEST EFFECT Studies show that diabetics benefit greatly from a diet high in fiber and complex carbohydrates. Patients with a low-fiber diet, especially if sugary foods are included, tend to experience rapid increases in blood-sugar levels. But foods such as whole-grain cereals, beans, and vegetables promote a slow, steady rise in blood sugar levels, allowing more effective control of diabetes.

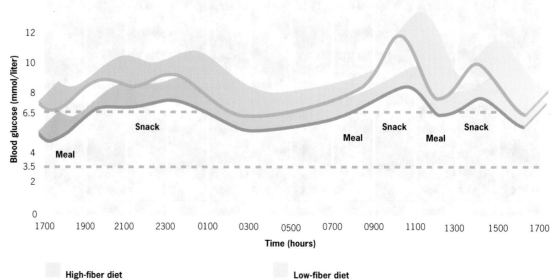

High-fiber diet   Low-fiber diet

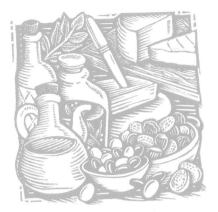

THE IMPORTANCE OF FATS

Fats, especially certain fatty acids, are vital to good health. They facilitate the absorption of fat-soluble vitamins, are involved in producing hormones, help support and protect vital organs, and insulate the body from cold. Fats are also an excellent source of energy. But heavy consumption of foods high in saturated fat has been linked to heart disease and some kinds of cancer. Nutritionists recommend that saturated fat be limited to no more than 10 percent of daily calories.

A VITAL NUTRIENT

The human body cannot function without fat. But it's important to know which types of fats and oils are more healthful, which can be harmful, and how much fat is optimal in the diet.

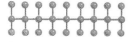

Saturated fatty acid

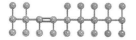

Monounsaturated fatty acid

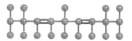

Polyunsaturated fatty acid

● **Hydrogen** atoms
◎ **Carbon** atoms

SATURATION LEVELS
The number of hydrogen atoms a fatty acid chain holds determines its level of saturation. A saturated fatty acid chain carries a full set of hydrogen atoms, which makes it harder to break up in the body. Saturated fats are major culprits in heart disease. In monounsaturated fats only one pair of atoms is missing, while in polyunsaturated fats two or more pairs are missing. These fats help to decrease the risk of heart disease.

Not all fats are created alike or equal; some are responsible for clogging arteries and they contribute to heart disease and stroke; others decrease the risk of blocked arteries.

At one time people commonly drank their coffee with cream, breakfasted on bacon, eggs, and buttered toast, and then ate a lunch consisting of a meat sandwich, a glass of whole milk, and a slice of pie with ice cream. Dinner consisted of more meat, at least two vegetables and another dessert. Vegetables were covered in butter, potatoes were fried, and very often the meat was beef, preferably well marbled and served with a gravy made from pan drippings.

Today this diet reads like a recipe for a heart attack, as all of these foods contain fat, and fatty foods have become the forbidden fruits of modern eating. Fat has become unpopular as a result of the many studies that have shown a link between dietary fat and heart disease. Although as yet controversial, evidence also seems to show a link between a fatty diet and some cancers, particularly those of the breast, bowel, and pancreas. Since heart disease and cancer are the leading causes of death for adults in the developed world, excess dietary fat is considered a health hazard. But this is not to say that all fats are bad for you. In fact, a diet that contains no fat can be just as dangerous as one that contains too much.

The human body could not function without fat. Every cell in the body contains fatty substances in its membranes. Fats also help the body to produce many hormones, some of which are related to fertility, while fat stored around the body's organs helps

---

FATS IN FOODS

A wide range of foods contains fat, and almost all foods contain more than one single type. Highest in saturated fats are meat and dairy products. The fattiest parts are the streaks or layers of visible fat on meat and the skin of chickens and other poultry. Processed foods such as potato chips, crackers, cookies, and ready-made meals, as well as cakes and pies, usually contain large amounts of fat, much of which is saturated.

Polyunsaturated and monounsaturated fats are found in fish, nuts, and seeds. Even olive oil, which is mainly monounsaturated fat, contains 14 percent saturated fat (see chart on page 52).

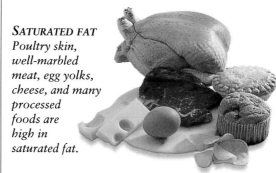

SATURATED FAT
Poultry skin, well-marbled meat, egg yolks, cheese, and many processed foods are high in saturated fat.

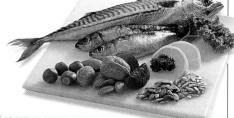

UNSATURATED FATS
Mackerel, sardines, nuts, and seeds provide polyunsaturated fat. Olive and canola oils are high in monounsaturated fat.

IS BUTTER BETTER THAN MARGARINE?

For years experts said that unsaturated fats, such as corn oil, were healthier than saturated fats, such as butter. Based on this advice, many people switched from butter to margarine made with corn oil, believing that it was a healthier alternative. But when liquid vegetable oils are made into solids such as margarine and shortening by the chemical process called

hydrogenation, some of the fats in the oil are changed into substances called trans fatty acids. New evidence suggests that these are, in fact, as harmful as, if not more than, saturated fats.

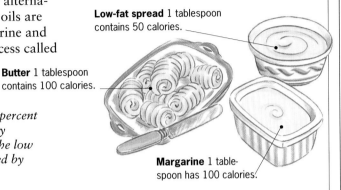

Low-fat spread 1 tablespoon contains 50 calories.

Butter 1 tablespoon contains 100 calories.

Margarine 1 table-spoon has 100 calories.

SPREADING FAT
Butter and margarine are both 81 percent fat. Low-fat spreads, however, may contain as little as 5 percent fat. The low percentage of fat is usually achieved by adding water to the spread.

to support and to protect them. The fat layer under the skin acts as a kind of thermal blanket that helps to keep the body warm. Furthermore, fats are an excellent source of energy, storable for future use.

The body can manufacture most types of fat from excess calories eaten in the form of carbohydrates and proteins, but it cannot manufacture them all. Two substances that scientists call essential fatty acids must come from the foods you eat. These two—linoleic acid and linolenic acid—occur naturally in some vegetable oils, seeds, and nuts. They make up the membranes of each of the trillions of cells in the body and are essential for the synthesis of hormonelike substances called prostaglandins.

If you are to stay healthy, you need to understand more about how fatty foods work in the body, the different types of fats that are found in food and which foods contain them. Then you will be able to choose the kinds of foods that will benefit your body and avoid those that could cause you problems.

THE DIFFERENT FATS
All fats contain fatty acids, which may be saturated or unsaturated. The difference lies in the types of molecules that make them up and the way that these molecules are arranged (see diagram, opposite). The molecules of a saturated fatty acid all contain a full complement of hydrogen atoms. This is what makes them "saturated." In contrast,

the molecules of unsaturated fatty acids have fewer hydrogen atoms. A high intake of saturated fats can lead to heart disease, but unsaturated fats have a protective effect.

It is possible to distinguish between saturated and unsaturated fats if you bear in mind that saturated fats, including saturated oils, are solid at room temperature, whereas unsaturated fats are liquid. Saturated fats are found mainly in animal products, such as meat and dairy foods, but also in tropical oils, for instance, palm oil, coconut oil, and cocoa butter.

Unsaturated fats occur in two forms, polyunsaturated and monounsaturated, and are found in vegetable oils. Olive, peanut, sesame, and canola oils contain mostly monounsaturated fats; corn, safflower, sunflower, soybean, and cottonseed oils are mainly made up of polyunsaturated fats. Polyunsaturated fats contain linoleic and linolenic acids, the essential fatty acids that cannot be made by the body.

HOW MUCH FAT DO YOU NEED?
To maintain optimal health, an adult needs a minimum amount of fat—30 grams per day—4 grams of which should contain the essential fatty acids found in polyunsaturated fats and oils. Thirty grams of fat per day may sound like a large amount but, in fact, it is far less than the daily intake of most people in the United States. Since every gram of fat provides 9 calories, 30 grams of fat amount to 270 calories,

Fat molecules
The majority of the body's fatty acids are large compounds called triglycerides: three fatty acids linked to a molecule of glycerol (an organic compound). The body's tissues assemble and disassemble triglycerides as needed.

Many triglycerides travel through the body and are stored in the fat depots, such as the upper arm and abdomen, until they are used for fuel.

Invisible fats
Unfortunately, much of the fat you eat is not visible. Foods like biscuits and pastries are loaded with "invisible" fats. To avoid these hidden fats, read the labels on packages before buying them. The fat content and the percentage of saturated fat should be clearly marked.

APPEALING LOOK
Manufacturers add fats to cookies and pastries to make them taste and look better. Coconut oil sprayed on crackers, for example, gives them a crisp outer coating and a glossy appearance.

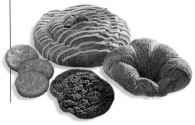

Garlic bread

To accompany a meal, forget butter-soaked garlic bread. Prepare this Mediterranean food the way the Italians do—with olive oil. Then add extra flavor with fresh herbs.

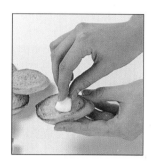

1 *Slice and lightly toast crusty French or Italian bread and rub the rough surfaces of the toast with a cut garlic clove.*

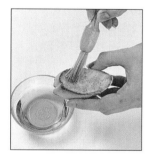

2 *Brush the bread on one side only with a little extra-virgin olive oil.*

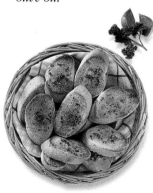

3 *Sprinkle herbs, for example, chopped fresh parsley, over the bread and serve.*

COMPARISON OF DIETARY FATS

The chart below shows the proportions of saturated, monounsaturated, and polyunsaturated fatty acids in various cooking fats. Also shown are the levels of linoleic and linolenic essential fatty acids, which are polyunsaturated fats.

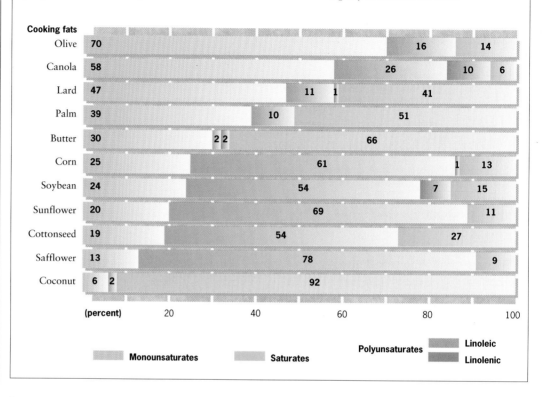

Cooking fats					
Olive	70			16	14
Canola	58		26	10	6
Lard	47	11	1	41	
Palm	39	10	51		
Butter	30	2	2	66	
Corn	25	61		1	13
Soybean	24	54	7	15	
Sunflower	20	69		11	
Cottonseed	19	54	27		
Safflower	13	78	9		
Coconut	6	2	92		

(percent) 20 40 60 80 100

Monounsaturates   Saturates   Polyunsaturates — Linoleic   Linolenic

between 13 and 14 percent of the average daily calorie intake for an adult (about 2,000 calories). However, the average adult in the United States gets about 42 percent of his or her calories from fat—about 840 calories a day. Most of these people, therefore, are eating almost three times as much fat as they need. Health authorities now recommend that fat intake be reduced to no more than 30 percent of calories, or about 600 calories per day, and of that total only 10 percent should be saturated fat.

HOW CAN YOU CUT DOWN ON FAT?

Easy ways to reduce fat in your diet are to trim all visible fat from meat, switch to low-fat or nonfat dairy foods, spread butter or margarine more thinly, and use cooking methods like steaming or broiling, instead of frying. You can further limit fat intake by eating smaller portions of meat, chicken, and high-fat cheese and other dairy products, and have them less often These foods are particularly high in saturated fats, the culprits of heart disease, stroke, and circu-latory disorders. If you cannot exclude meat completely from your life, use cooking techniques that promote removal of some of the fat. For instance, cook a meat-based sauce, soup, or stew a day ahead and refrigerate it overnight to allow fat to solidify at the top of the dish for easy removal.

Vegetarian diets are generally lower in fat than a standard regimen because they lack meat, which is high in fat, and feature vegetables and grains, which are low in fat. However, some vegetarians make up the difference by consuming many whole-milk dairy products. A dish of macaroni and cheese made with a sauce based on butter, whole milk, and Cheddar cheese, for example, can wreak as much havoc in fat count as a breakfast of bacon and eggs. A better way to obtain protein is by carefully combining vegetable sources (see page 31).

Selecting low-fat snack foods and desserts is also sensible. More manufacturers today are producing nonfat crackers and pretzels; baking, instead of frying, potato and corn chips; and making popcorn with low-fat coatings and cakes with very low or no fat.

However, it pays to read and interpret labels carefully. When a product is labeled 98 percent fat free, this figure may represent a percentage of the food's weight, rather than calories. For example, 2-percent milk contains 5 grams of fat. In a 1-cup serving this equals 45 calories from fat, or 38 percent of the 120 total calories. The labels of most processed foods today must state what percentage of calories come from fat.

EATING THE "GOOD" FATS

Another way to reduce your intake of saturated fats is to substitute monounsaturated olive oil or a polyunsaturated vegetable oil for butter, lard, and shortening in cooking and baking. Although they have as many calories as saturated oils, their effect on cholesterol metabolism—a factor in coronary artery disease—is different (see page 110).

(see page 110)

Certain fish oils are particularly beneficial. They contain a class of essential fatty acids known as omega-3 fatty acids, which are polyunsaturates that have been shown to lower cholesterol and reduce the blood's ability to clot and clog up the arteries. Cold-water ocean fish, such as mackerel, herring, tuna, sardines, and salmon, are all rich in this type of oil. Experts recommend that you eat these fish twice a week.

Can you eat too little fat?

Although many people believe that they are eating too much fat, some are actually not eating enough. Persons on strict weight-loss diets can be at risk of eating too little fat, as can those who eat a fat-restricted diet based heavily on complex carbohydrates. Everyone needs some fat (about 30 grams per day). Some experts believe that anorexia and bulimia sufferers may become infertile because they do not eat the fats necessary for normal hormone production.

Dietary recommendations for middle-aged people should not be applied to young children, who have high energy requirements and must have fat to meet their needs. A change to low-fat or nonfat products such as skim milk can mean that a child's hunger is satisfied before energy needs have been met. Children should drink whole milk until at least two years of age.

REDUCED-FAT EATING

HIGH FAT	HEALTHIER FAT
POTATOES	
Deep-fat frying	Cook "oven fries" with minimal oil. Blot fries on paper towels.
POULTRY	
Skin on Butter basted	Remove skin before cooking. Baste with stock.
MEAT	
Heavily marbled cuts Pan gravy	Choose lean cuts; trim fat off meat. Skim fat off gravy.
PASTA	
Served with meaty sauces or creamy sauces	Make vegetable-based sauces. Toss pasta in a little olive oil with herbs.
FISH	
Fried	Poach, bake, broil, steam, or microwave.
STEWS	
Meat-based	Trim fat off meat, skim fat off stew, use more vegetables and legumes. Use minimum fat or olive oil to sauté meat or vegetables.
CHEESE TOPPINGS	
Whole-milk cheese	Use low-fat cheese or bread crumb toppings flavored with herbs and garlic.
GARLIC BREAD	
Butter	Use olive oil; spread with pastry brush.

The Naturopath

Naturopathy is a system of primary health care that uses natural measures, particularly diet, to restore and promote the body's self-healing processes. Taking a holistic approach, a naturopath attempts to identify and treat the causes of illness.

Head
Ear and neck
Face
Lung
Mouth and throat
Chest
Upper back
Upper abdomen
Lower back
Lower abdomen
Pelvis

IRIS DIAGNOSIS
Some naturopaths use careful inspection of the eye as a diagnostic aid. The iris (the colored part of the eye) is believed to have reflex connections with other organs and tissues in the body. Changes in the texture of these zones may reveal information about the health of the related organs.

Naturopaths may advise or apply treatments that differ from those of conventional medicine but are nevertheless complementary to the services available from your doctor.

What sort of treatment does a naturopath give?
Instead of relying on drugs, naturopaths use various therapies to capitalize on the body's natural healing ability. Dietary therapy, fasting, hydrotherapy, massage, and homeopathy—one or several of these approaches may be used to treat an individual's ailment.

What sort of illnesses can a naturopath cure or alleviate?
Naturopaths treat a wide range of illnesses, both acute and chronic, as well as infections. For acute illnesses, such as colds, coughs, and gastroenteritis, a naturopath will suggest safe and effective ways of relieving the symptoms without resorting to antibiotics or other suppressive drugs. A naturopath will apply similar treatments to alleviate chronic illnesses, such as rheumatism, arthritis, and asthma.

Why would I consult a naturopath?
If you want to take more personal responsibility for your health and prefer to use natural treatments whenever possible, you might decide to seek the advice of a naturopath.

The naturopath tailors his advice to your individual needs and will usually suggest modifications to your diet for a few days in conjunction with other treatments such as compresses or herbal remedies.

How does a naturopath decide which treatment to give?
At your first visit the naturopath will ask you about any health problems, your diet, work, exercise, lifestyle, and personal history. All these elements will be taken into consideration when establishing your health program.

The naturopath is trained in basic medical sciences, such as anatomy, physiology, and diagnosis. This training enables him to carry out a physical examination and to use

Origins

Although the term *naturopathy* was not adopted until the end of the 19th century, this system of medicine dates back to Hippocrates, whose recommendations more than 2,000 years ago included the maxim "Let food be your medicine and let your medicine be your food."

In the 19th and early 20th centuries, pioneers such as Henry Lindlahr in the United States, Max Bircher-Benner in Switzerland, and Stanley Lief in England all ran residential clinics at which patients were able to fast and undergo physical therapy and water treatments to tackle a wide variety of ailments. These forerunners of modern scientific naturopathy were determined advocates of diets low in

fats, salt, and refined foods—diets that are now widely endorsed by health experts around the world.

FATHER OF WESTERN MEDICINE
The Greek physician Hippocrates (c.460–c.370 B.C.) maintained that the body could heal itself with natural cures, such as a good diet.

the information gained from the initial consultation not only for normal diagnostic purposes but also to assess your vitality and potential for better health. Many naturopaths also use other investigations, such as blood, sweat, and hair analysis, to check your levels of the minerals and trace elements that are essential for a healthy body. Some naturopaths may also use iris diagnosis (see opposite).

How does naturopathy help infectious diseases?

Naturopaths regard many acute illnesses, especially those accompanied by fever, as an indication of the self-healing mechanisms at work. As your immune system starts to overcome the infection, your body temperature rises, either locally with inflammation or more generally with a fever. This must be allowed to take its course without suppressing the symptoms. One of the most effective treatments in this situation is fasting or, in cases where this may not be appropriate, a restricted diet, such as fresh fruit only for two or three days. This allows your body to rid itself of the toxic compounds associated with the infection. You may also be advised on how to use cold compresses and other forms of hydrotherapy to assist detoxification, regulate temperature, and increase your immune response. Some naturopaths may also prescribe herbal medicines to aid recovery.

How does naturopathy help chronic diseases?

When chronic degenerative diseases such as arthritis have taken their toll, the body's self-healing capacity may be limited, but naturopathic treatment can still help to keep the patient more comfortable and reduce the sufferer's dependence on pain-relieving drugs. Diet control is often a major part of this management.

For patients with heart and circulatory conditions, the naturopath is able to give guidance on how to substitute unsaturated fats in the diet for those that are not easily digested. Advice on exercise and relaxation is also important for dealing with these disorders.

How can I find a naturopath?

You may consult a naturopath without referral from a medical practitioner, although it is preferable that your doctor know that you are seeking such advice.

Most naturopaths are in private practice and may be seen by appointment. Some practitioners work in residential clinics where a range of treatments, such as spa baths, is available to patients.

In the United States the majority of naturopaths belong to the American Association of Naturopathic Physicians at P.O. Box 20386, Seattle, WA 98102.

WHAT YOU CAN DO AT HOME

Nearly everyone experiences an attack of vomiting and diarrhea at some time. This may be caused by tainted food or gastric "flu." In either case, the following diet may help (seek the advice of your general practitioner before undertaking this diet if you have any medical disorder, such as diabetes or epilepsy).

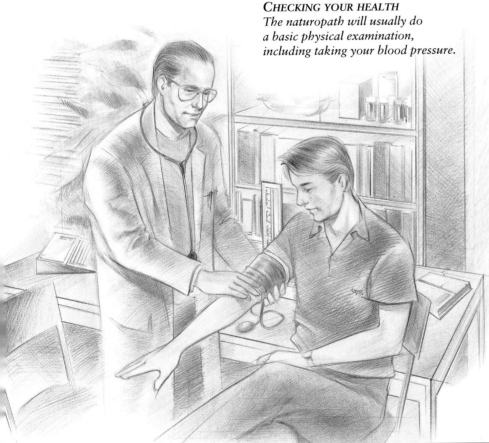

CHECKING YOUR HEALTH
The naturopath will usually do a basic physical examination, including taking your blood pressure.

TIME	DIET
First 24 hours	Drink one glass of unsweetened apple juice or mineral water every two or three hours. This allows the stomach and intestines to clear fermented matter and irritants.
Second day	Breakfast—a little low-fat yogurt. Lunch—a dish of finely grated or pureed apple. Evening meal—if you feel better, a bowl of vegetable soup.
Third day	Fruit and yogurt for breakfast; soup or steamed vegetables with a dish of brown rice for lunch and dinner.

THE DANGERS OF A HIGH-FAT DIET

Many international studies have indicated that there is a link between high-fat diets and increased death rates from hypertension, heart disease, stroke, and some types of cancer.

Foods that elevate cholesterol

Despite all the attention that cholesterol has received, many people still do not know which foods contain the fats that produce it.

Cholesterol-elevating saturated fats are found mainly in foods derived from animals—meat, poultry, shellfish, and dairy products. Coconut and palm oils, although derived from plants, are also high in saturated fats. Only 10 percent of your fat calories should come from saturated fats.

HIGH-FAT FOODS
A high intake of whole-milk dairy products and fatty meats will raise your level of "bad" cholesterol—LDLs—and increase your risk of heart disease. But a fatty food like avocado provides unsaturated fat, which does not harm the arteries.

The connection between a high-fat diet and life-threatening diseases such as hypertension, heart disease, stroke, and cancer centers on a waxy substance called cholesterol. Although naturally occurring cholesterol is found in some foods, particularly organ meats and egg yolks, most of the cholesterol in the body is manufactured in the liver and other tissues from ingested saturated fats.

There are three different types of lipoprotein in the bloodstream that are responsible for transporting cholesterol throughout the body. Two of these lipoproteins are harmful if excessive, while the third seems to have a beneficial effect on your arteries.

Low-density lipoprotein (LDL) and very-low-density lipoprotein (VLDL) tend to stick to the lining of the arteries and appear to be directly related to the amount of saturated fat a person eats. However, high-density lipoprotein (HDL) has the capacity to dissolve existing cholesterol residue in the arteries and scrub it from the blood vessel walls as it passes. Levels of protective HDL cholesterol are increased by a low-fat diet that contains a good supply of fruit and veg-

etables. Other factors that increase this "good" cholesterol are exercising regularly, drinking small quantities of alcohol, particularly red wine, and eating cold-water fish such as tuna, salmon, herring, or mackerel, which are rich in omega-3 fatty acids.

CHOLESTEROL AND DISEASE

When people eat more saturated fats than they need, cholesterol production within the body increases, and excess cholesterol ends up in the bloodstream, where it accumulates in the walls of the arteries.

Over time the arterial walls can become lined with these fatty deposits, or plaque. This condition—a thickening and stiffening of the walls of the arteries—is known as atherosclerosis. The thicker walls mean that the passageway for blood is narrower—which increases blood pressure.

High blood pressure, or hypertension, is a major health risk. When arteries are narrowed, blood must be pushed more forcefully through them, placing the walls under additional strain. They can begin to weaken and form bulges, known as aneurisms. If any of these bulges rupture, they may cause

HIGH FAT AND CANCER

Cancer is a complex disease with many causes, but certain types have been associated with diet. Bile acids in the colon that can turn cells cancerous are stimulated by fat. Fat is also known to act as a fuel that promotes tumor growth. Recent research indicates that eating too much fat can depress the immune system's tumor surveillance mechanism.

Despite these findings, the evidence remains controversial and the link between diet and cancer is yet to be completely proven. Some scientists now believe that oxidized fat and cholesterol may be the culprits and that high levels of natural antioxidants (see page 94), present in fruits, vegetables, and vegetable oils, may play a protective role.

High Blood Cholesterol

Cholesterol is a normal component of blood, but when blood-cholesterol levels are permanently raised, the individual becomes susceptible to a number of diseases. A high cholesterol level may be caused by various factors, among them poor diet, alcohol abuse, and genetic disease. Sufferers may need to make several modifications to their diet to control this condition.

At the age of 40, Barbara Becker spends most of her time caring for her husband and two teenage sons. Recently, she noticed some little yellowish white patches on her eyelids, which prompted her to go see her doctor. She learned that these spots, fatty deposits called xanthomas, are harmless in themselves, but that they can be indicators of dangerously high blood cholesterol levels. Her doctor explained that continuously high cholesterol levels contribute to heart disease, high blood pressure, and stroke. However, through a low-fat diet, proper medication, and giving up cigarettes, she can control her cholesterol. He also said that her form of high cholesterol is usually inherited. Normally, there are no visible signs of high cholesterol; only a blood test will reveal the level.

WHAT BARBARA SHOULD DO
Barbara and her doctor should work out a diet that will help her to reduce her intake of saturated fats and cholesterol and increase her intake of soluble fiber (see page 46). She not only needs to learn about low-fat food selection and cooking methods, but also to teach those around her about the risks of poor eating habits, at home as well as outside of it.

Barbara must take the medication prescribed by her doctor to control blood cholesterol levels, and have regular checkups. She should also encourage her sons to have their cholesterol levels checked at least once every five years, in case they have inherited her condition.

Behavior-modification techniques can help Barbara to give up smoking. Her doctor or a local hospital may provide advice.

Action Plan

HEALTH
Seek advice on a changed dietary pattern. Go for more regular checkups. Stop smoking now.

FAMILY
Make sure the boys' cholesterol levels are tested. Also try to get the whole family more involved in their health and educate them about eating more healthfully.

HOW THINGS TURN OUT FOR BARBARA

Barbara's doctor referred her to a dietitian, who assessed her current eating pattern and lifestyle. She recommended a balanced, reduced-fat diet with several servings of fruit and vegetables every day to help Barbara eat more healthfully. Barbara's improved diet gave her more energy, but she has gone back to preparing and eating more of the quick foods and frozen meals her family enjoys. She finds this worrisome because the boys' cholesterol levels did turn out to be higher than normal. Another trip to the dietitian has been planned, this time with the boys, to get more ideas about changing their diet. Smoking is still a problem, but Barbara is now down to three cigarettes a day.

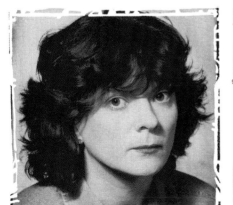

HEALTH
A diet high in saturated fats and a lifelong addiction to cigarettes have added to the risks already existing with an inherited tendency toward high cholesterol levels.

FAMILY
A genetic disposition to high levels of cholesterol may have been inherited by a sufferer's children as well as herself.

LOWERING CHOLESTEROL LEVELS

Changing the types of foods you eat can help you to keep your overall cholesterol levels low or reduce them if they have become too high and can raise the levels of "good" cholesterol—HDLs.

▶ *Increase the amount of fruits and vegetables in your diet, whether fresh, frozen, or canned.*

▶ *Eat more foods containing water-soluble fiber, such as legumes and oat bran (see page 46).*

BENEFICIAL FOODS
Salmon, legumes, fruits, vegetables, and red wine actually lower "bad" cholesterol and reduce the blood's ability to clot and clog up the arteries.

a stroke or cardiac arrest. Strokes occur when arteries in the brain rupture, leaking blood into the surrounding tissue, whereas the heart may stop if its blood supply is interfered with. Even if such severe consequences do not occur, high blood pressure can cause damage to the kidneys or retina.

Large-scale international studies connecting eating habits with patterns of illness have tended to confirm the link between a diet high in saturated fat and heart disease. In Japan and the Mediterranean countries people follow a diet low in saturated fat, and they are less likely to develop heart disease than citizens of North American or northern European countries, who eat higher amounts of saturated fat. They also consume more fish, which is low in saturated fat, and less meat. In the Mediterranean countries people do eat a high amount of fat, but it is mainly olive oil, not butter.

The health and eating habits of the Inuits of Greenland confirm the importance of the type of fat eaten. Although the Inuits eat a very-high-fat diet, heart disease and stroke are virtually unknown. The reason for this anomaly is that the fats they eat come from fatty fish and seal blubber and are mostly unsaturated. These foods also contain large amounts of omega-3 fatty acids, which lower levels of "bad" cholesterol (LDLs), dilate the blood vessels (which helps to relieve pressure), and counteract the clumping of blood platelets.

International studies have also shown a high correlation between the incidence of breast cancer and the level of dietary fat. In Europe and

LOW FAT OR LOW CALORIE?

Reports concerning the links between dietary fat and major illnesses have stimulated considerable public demand for foods containing little or no fat, particularly among dieters. But fat-free products do not guarantee weight loss, and if they form too large a part of your diet, they may even be harmful.

Fat-free products can help you to lose weight only if you are eating fewer calories than you burn up. Being fat free is not the same as being calorie free. Carbohydrates and proteins in food contain calories, and eating excessive amounts of fat-free foods in the mistaken belief that they will not make you fat will certainly not help to make you slim.

Even if you are dieting, you should be sure to eat some fats or oils every day. Dressing salads with a little olive oil, adding seeds and soybean products to your meals, and eating oily fish two or three times a week may cost you some calories, but they are a good investment for long-term health.

North America, where the percentage of fat in the diet is high, the rate of breast cancer is also high; in Japan and other countries where less fat is eaten, the rates for this type of cancer are lower.

Colorectal cancer is also most prevalent in economically developed countries, where many individuals eat a diet that is high in fat and low in fiber.

LOWER-FAT SUBSTITUTES

USE	INSTEAD OF	SAVE
2 egg whites	1 whole egg	5 g fat
1 oz part-skim-milk mozzarella	1 oz Cheddar cheese	4 g fat
1 oz cottage cheese	1 oz cream cheese	9 g fat
1 tbsp evaporated skim milk	1 tbsp whipping cream	5 g fat
1 oz extra-lean roast ham	1 oz hard salami	12 g fat
1 chicken frankfurter	1 beef frankfurter	4 g fat
4 oz tuna in water	4 oz tuna in oil	8 g fat
1 4-oz baked potato	1 3½-oz serving potato chips	10 g fat
1 banana	1 frosted doughnut	13 g fat
2 oz sorbet	2 oz ice cream	10 g fat

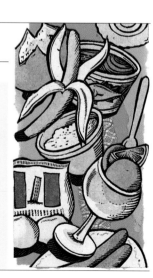

CHAPTER 5

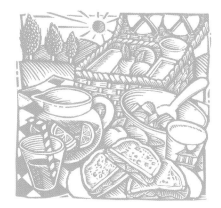

VITAMINS AND MINERALS

Although needed by the body in only tiny amounts, vitamins and minerals are essential for good health. A balanced diet can provide ample amounts of these essential nutrients, but poor eating habits can deprive you of the vitamins and minerals you need. Supplements may make up some of the difference. In the long run, however, it's much better to eat sensibly, choose foods wisely, and prepare, cook, and store them properly.

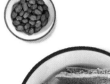

Peanuts—1½ oz contain 6 mg of niacin.

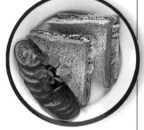

A tuna sandwich contains 6 mg of niacin.

SOURCES OF NIACIN (VITAMIN B₃)
A sandwich containing 1 oz of tuna provides as much of the B vitamin niacin as 1½ oz of peanuts.

MICRONUTRIENTS

Vitamins are life-sustaining substances that humans need to keep their bodies running smoothly. Minerals have an equally vital role in developing and maintaining the body's functions.

Unlike the macronutrients—proteins, carbohydrates, and fats—vitamins do not provide energy or serve as building materials. They enable the body to function efficiently by regulating biochemical processes such as growth, metabolism, cellular reproduction, digestion, and the oxidation of blood.

There are 13 recognized vitamins, and these are classified into two groups, water soluble and fat soluble. Water-soluble vitamins, which include the B-complex group and C, remain for no more than three days in various body tissues; therefore, they need to be replenished daily. They are absorbed through the intestines into the bloodstream, and any excess that the body does not need passes out in urine. If your diet is severely lacking in these vitamins, deficiency symptoms can occur within weeks.

The four fat-soluble vitamins—A, D, E, and K—are absorbed through the intestine with dietary fats and (except vitamin K) are stored in the liver and fatty tissue. They can be stockpiled for periods that, depending on quantity, can be as long as a year (or more in the case of vitamin A), so you do not need to consume large quantities of them every day. In fact, excessive amounts of fat-soluble vitamins in the diet can be harmful.

THE ROLE OF THE LIVER

The liver, which produces bile, a digestive juice, plays an active role in breaking down fats in foods. This allows fat-soluble vitamins and other nutrients to be absorbed through the intestine, converting them for use in the body.

The liver is also a storehouse for nutrients, such as minerals and three of the fat-soluble vitamins: A, D, and E.

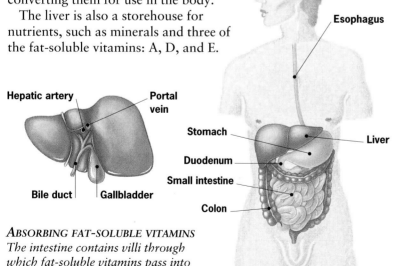

Hepatic artery
Portal vein
Esophagus
Stomach
Liver
Duodenum
Small intestine
Colon
Bile duct
Gallbladder

ABSORBING FAT-SOLUBLE VITAMINS
The intestine contains villi through which fat-soluble vitamins pass into the bloodstream. Excess vitamins are carried to the liver for storage.

WATER-SOLUBLE VITAMINS

There are eight members of the B-complex group. Each has separate functions, but they all are essential for efficient metabolism—the process by which the body converts food into tissue or uses it to produce energy. B vitamins play a major role in the body's production of energy, working with enzymes—body substances that break down foods—to convert carbohydrates and fats into fuel for the body. They are also necessary for the smooth functioning of the nervous and immune systems.

Vitamin B₁ (thiamine) aids the release of energy from food and from all body cells, including the brain and nerve cells, and the muscles. Vitamin B₂ (riboflavin) helps to liberate energy from carbohydrates and fats.

Vitamin B₃ (niacin) is also crucial for energy release and protein metabolism—conversion of protein to substances of use to the body—and the production of certain hormones. Unlike thiamine and riboflavin, which can be obtained only from food, niacin can be partially synthesized within the body from the amino acid tryptophan. Since not enough can be made, however, dietary sources are also needed.

B₁₂ AND THE INTRINSIC FACTOR

Cells in the stomach lining secrete an enzyme called the intrinsic factor. This binds with vitamin B₁₂, allowing it to be absorbed into the bloodstream from the intestinal tract.

People who lack this enzyme must have vitamin B₁₂ injected into the bloodstream under the supervision of a doctor or clinical nutritionist.

THE STOMACH

The wall of the stomach consists of three layers of smooth muscle. Its inner lining is made up of cells that secrete gastric juice, which contains the intrinsic factor.

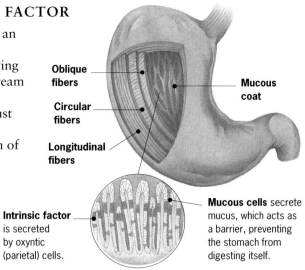

Oblique fibers

Circular fibers

Longitudinal fibers

Mucous coat

Intrinsic factor is secreted by oxyntic (parietal) cells.

Mucous cells secrete mucus, which acts as a barrier, preventing the stomach from digesting itself.

PRESERVING VITAMINS

Vitamins are very fragile nutrients that are easily destroyed during storage and cooking. Here are a few tips to help you get the most from food.

▶ *Store foods in a cool, dark area because light accelerates vitamin loss, particularly of vitamins A, D, and B₂.*

▶ *Rinse fruit and vegetables under cold running water. Do not soak them because the vitamins will leach into the water.*

▶ *Microwave, pressure-cook, or steam vegetables in a small amount of water. Some of the vitamins will pass into the cooking water and will be lost unless the water is utilized.*

Pantothenic acid, another member of the B group, also enables the body to obtain energy from foods and to manufacture some important hormones as well.

Vitamin B₆ (pyridoxine) helps the body to absorb and use proteins. The more high-protein foods you eat, such as meat, the more foods containing vitamin B₆ you will need. Vitamin B₆ also helps to maintain the central nervous system and, along with folic acid and B₁₂, helps to form hemoglobin, the oxygen-carrying pigment in red blood cells. The metabolism of essential fatty acids (see page 51) is another role key for vitamin B₆ and it is involved in more than 80 different biochemical reactions as well.

Vitamin B₁₂ is essential for healthy red blood cells and for preventing or relieving anemia. In the manufacture of red blood cells, vitamin B₁₂ acts in conjunction with folic acid; both of which play a vital part in the synthesis of genetic material. It also helps the nervous system function smoothly and assists in metabolism of amino acids. The only natural sources of B₁₂ are animal products. People who eat no meat, dairy, eggs, or fish need foods fortified with B₁₂.

Biotin, another water-soluble vitamin, helps the body to utilize essential fatty acids and is necessary for releasing energy from carbohydrates and proteins as well as fat.

Vitamin C

Vitamin C (ascorbic acid) plays a major role in healing wounds and burns and it aids in the absorption of iron from grains and leafy vegetables. Vitamin C helps to produce collagen, a major component of the connective tissue that holds the various structures of the body together. Contrary to popular belief, studies have not yet supported the claim that large doses of vitamin C can completely ward off or cure the common cold. Research suggests, however, that it does help to reduce the cold's duration. Vitamin C is also a potent antioxidant, neu-

---

NUTRIENT COMBINATIONS

Particular vitamins and minerals eaten in tandem will work more effectively in the body. Some are found in one food alone, others in combinations of foods.

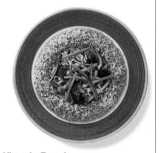

Vitamin D and calcium— the flesh of sardines contains vitamin D, and their bones calcium. A good level of vitamin D aids the body to use calcium more effectively.

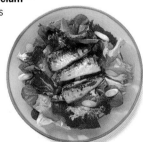

Vitamin E and essential fatty acids— sunflower seeds add vitamin E, which protects against oxidation of essential fatty acids provided by the olive oil in a stir-fry.

Vitamin B₁₂ and folic acid— a good source of vitamin B₁₂, eggs can be combined with spinach, rich in folic acid, to form new cells in the body.

Vitamin C and iron— tomato sauce provides vitamin C, which helps in the absorption of iron from rice and vegetables.

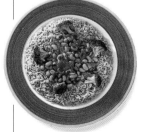

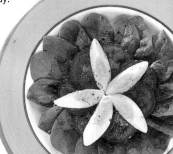

An orange
contains 54 mg
of calcium.

Milk—1 cup (8 fl oz)
contains 297 mg
of calcium.

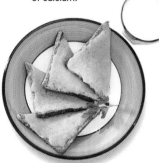

SOURCES OF CALCIUM
You can meet 70 percent
of your daily calcium
needs by drinking an
8-fl-oz glass of milk
and eating two slices of
whole-grain toast, 1 oz
of cheese, and an orange.

tralizing free radicals. These are unstable molecules that, if unchecked, contribute to heart disease and cancers, and are associated with the aging process (see page 94). It has also been demonstrated that vitamin C helps to block the formation of cancer-causing substances called nitrosamines, which are formed in the stomach from nitrites in foods.

FAT-SOLUBLE VITAMINS

Vitamin A (retinol) is essential for good vision and for the manufacture of a light-sensitive pigment in the retina called rhodopsin, or visual purple. It also helps to form healthy skin and mucous membranes, such as the linings of the nose and digestive system, and is essential for the proper functioning of the liver. Growth and development also rely on an adequate intake of vitamin A.

Beta carotene, which is converted into vitamin A in the body, is a powerful antioxidant, mopping up free radicals before damage can occur. Carotenes received the name because they were first isolated from carrots. About

35 of more than 6,000 carotenes in nature can be partially converted by the body in the intestinal wall to vitamin A. The remainder are absorbed directly into the body.

Vitamin D (cholecalciferol) is vital for the development and maintenance of bones and teeth and aids in the absorption and metabolism of calcium and phosphorus. Nicknamed the sunshine vitamin, it is made by the skin when the skin is exposed to the ultraviolet light in sunshine. It is also found in a number of foods, particularly fortified milk.

Vitamin E (tocopherol) is a potent antioxidant. Along with vitamin C and the carotenes, it is important for dissipating free radicals (see page 94) and protecting the essential fatty acids from oxidation. Recent research suggests that vitamin E helps to protect against cancer and heart disease by limiting the production of free radicals.

Vitamin K is essential for producing substances in the liver that promote blood clotting. It is found in a wide range of foods, and because it is also made by intestinal

RECOMMENDED DAILY ALLOWANCE OF VITAMINS

AGES	A μg	D μg	C mg	B_1 mg	B_2 mg	B_3 mg	B_6 mg	FOLIC ACID μg	B_{12} μg
INFANTS									
6 mo	375	7.5	30	0.3	0.4	5	0.3	25	0.3
6 mo–1 yr	375	10	35	0.4	0.5	6	0.6	35	0.5
CHILDREN									
1–3 yr	400	10	40	0.7	0.8	9	1.0	50	0.7
4–6	500	10	45	0.9	1.1	12	1.1	75	1.0
7–10	700	10	45	1.0	1.2	13	1.4	100	1.4
MALES									
11–14	1,000	10	50	1.3	1.5	17	1.7	150	2.0
15–18	1,000	10	60	1.5	1.8	20	2.0	200	2.0
19–24	1,000	10	60	1.5	1.7	19	2.0	200	2.0
25–50	1,000	5	60	1.5	1.7	19	2.0	200	2.0
51 & over	1,000	5	60	1.2	1.4	15	2.0	200	2.0
FEMALES									
11–14	800	10	50	1.1	1.3	15	1.4	150	2.0
15–18	800	10	60	1.1	1.3	15	1.5	180	2.0
19–24	800	10	60	1.1	1.3	15	1.6	180	2.0
25–50	800	5	60	1.1	1.3	15	1.6	180	2.0
51 & over	800	5	60	1.0	1.2	13	1.6	180	2.0
Pregnant	800	10	70	1.5	1.6	17	2.2	400	2.2
Nursing	1,300	10	95	1.6	1.8	20	2.1	280	2.6

mg= milligrams   µg= micrograms

bacteria, most people have some supply. Newborn babies, however, are born with low stores of the vitamin and are at risk of hemorrhaging. Vitamin K is now routinely administered to infants.

THE MINERALS

Like vitamins, minerals are vital for the body's well-being—they are essential components of critical enzymes that help the body to break down food.

Calcium, phosphorus, magnesium, potassium, sodium, and chloride are known as macrominerals; they are needed in fairly large quantities by the body.

Calcium is indispensable for building and maintaining strong bones and teeth. In fact, about 99 percent of the body's calcium is found in the bones and teeth, with the remaining 1 percent being distributed in the cells, blood, and bodily fluids. Everybody needs a good supply of calcium throughout life to sustain bone density and strength, but the greater the bone mass that is laid down

early in life, the less risk there is of bones becoming porous in old age (see page 69).

The calcium in cells performs a variety of functions, including ensuring the proper functioning of the nerves and muscles and normal clotting of the blood. Vitamin D is required for calcium absorption, but studies have shown that exercising will also speed up this process.

Magnesium is essential for the proper functioning of nerves and muscles and for maintaining bone structure. It also aids fat metabolism, regulation of body temperature, and protein synthesis.

Phosphorus works closely with calcium and magnesium to build and maintain bones and teeth. It also plays a role in releasing energy from carbohydrates and transporting fats around the body.

Potassium, one of the body's most abundant minerals, is crucial for controlling water balance in the body's tissues and cells. It also helps to regulate blood pressure.

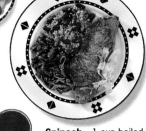

Strawberries—2 cups provide 1.2 mg of iron.

Spinach—1 cup boiled provides 4 mg of iron.

Cranberry juice—8 fl oz supplies 0.4 mg of iron.

SOURCES OF IRON
A meal consisting of a 4-oz steak, 3½ oz of red kidney beans, and the same amount of spinach and bulgur wheat, plus 5 oz of strawberries and a glass of cranberry juice supplies 12 mg of iron.

RECOMMENDED DAILY ALLOWANCE OF MINERALS

AGES	CALCIUM mg	PHOSPHORUS mg	MAGNESIUM mg	IRON mg	ZINC mg	IODINE µg
INFANTS						
6 mo	400	300	40	6	5	40
6 mo–1 yr	600	500	60	10	5	50
CHILDREN						
1–3 yr	800	800	80	10	10	70
4–6	800	800	120	10	10	90
7–10	800	800	170	10	10	120
MALES						
11–14	1,200	1,200	270	12	15	150
15–18	1,200	1,200	400	12	15	150
19–24	1,200	1,200	350	10	15	150
25–50	800	800	350	10	15	150
51 & over	800	800	350	10	15	150
FEMALES						
11–14	1,200	1,200	280	15	12	150
15–18	1,200	1,200	300	15	12	150
19–24	1,200	1,200	280	15	12	150
25–50	800	800	280	15	12	150
51 & over	800	800	280	10	12	150
Pregnant	1,200	1,200	320	30	15	175
Nursing	1,200	1,200	355	15	19	200

mg= milligrams   µg= micrograms

Sodium and chloride work as partners with potassium to balance the body's fluids. Sodium is also essential for nerve activity.

Iron, zinc, iodine, manganese, selenium, chromium, copper, and fluoride are all trace elements. Although the body needs smaller amounts of these minerals than it does of the macrominerals, they have an equally vital role in the functioning of the body.

Iron is essential for the formation of hemoglobin, the red pigment in the bloodstream that transports oxygen from the lungs to all the cells of the body. It is also an important component of many enzymes.

Zinc is necessary for normal mental, physical, and reproductive development, hair and skin growth, wound healing, and insulin production.

VITAMINS—SOURCES AND EFFECTS

There are many tales about the wonderful effects that vitamins can have—and some of them are true. Other claims exaggerate and expand upon the properties of vitamins until we no longer know if a carrot will help us to see in the dark. The table below should help you discern the difference between myth and reality.

VITA	SOURCES	SAID TO	ACTUALLY IS/DOES
A	Liver, fish (cod and halibut), eggs, dairy products, green and orange vegetables.	Give superhuman sight. Cure cancer. Preserve youthful looks.	Vital to good vision. Important for healthy skin and immunity.
B$_1$	Wheat germ, pork and other lean meats, milk, eggs, yeast, dried beans.	Prevent fatigue. Cure depression.	Necessary for functioning of brain, nerve cells, and heart.
B$_2$	Milk, dairy products, eggs, meats, leafy green vegetables, nuts, liver.	Improve vision. Cure baldness.	Required to release energy from foods.
B$_3$	Peanuts, poultry, lean meats, milk, eggs, whole grains, liver.	Help schizophrenia. Cure depression.	Maintain healthy skin, nerves, and digestive system.
PANTO-THENIC ACID	Eggs, dairy products, fish, cereals, dried peas and beans, brewer's yeast.	Ease stress. Return gray hair to normal. Ease allergies.	Essential in the synthesis of many body materials.
B$_6$	Bananas, whole-grain breads, meats, eggs, dried beans, nuts, chicken, fish, liver.	Help arthritis. Relieve nausea. Act as a tranquilizer. Relieve nervous or muscle disorders.	Important in chemical reactions between proteins and amino acids. Aid formation of red blood cells.
B$_{12}$	Eggs, shellfish, meats, milk, poultry.	Cure nervous disorders.	Develop red blood cells and maintain the nervous system.
BIOTIN	Eggs, dairy products, liver, cereals.	Help muscle pain. Help cure baldness and dermatitis.	Help to metabolize amino acids, carbohydrates, and fats.
FOLIC ACID	Leafy green vegetables, dried peas and beans, liver, yeast.	Alleviate mental illness. Prevent birth defects. Cure anemia.	Act with B$_{12}$ to produce hemoglobin. Important in DNA synthesis. Prevent neural tube defects (spina bifida).
C	Citrus fruits, strawberries, black currants, tomatoes, melons, potatoes, bell peppers.	Cure allergies. Cure arthritis. Cure and prevent colds. Prevent atherosclerosis. Prevent certain cancers.	Promote healthy gums, teeth, and connective tissue. Aid the healing of wounds. Fight free radicals. Strengthen immune system.
D	Cod liver oil, oily fish, egg yolks, fortified milk, and margarines.	Cure arthritis.	Promote strong bones and teeth. Prevent rickets and osteomalacia (softening of bones).
E	Vegetable oils, sunflower seeds, nuts, wheat germ, leafy green vegetables.	Improve virility and stamina. Heal burns and scars. Prevent aging.	Protect tissue against oxidative damage.
K	Leafy green vegetables, soybeans, cereals.		Necessary for normal blood clotting.

Iodine is vital for normal functioning of the thyroid gland, which regulates metabolism, the rate at which the body releases energy from food. The mineral also helps to maintain healthy skin, hair, and nails.

Manganese aids reproduction, cell function, and bone growth and development. Selenium is an important antioxidant and functions as such in cooperation with vitamins A, C, and E. Chromium maintains normal blood sugar levels and is essential for insulin to act properly.

Copper is needed in small quantities by the body to develop red blood cells and facilitate bone synthesis.

Fluoride is vital for the formation and strength of bones and teeth, hardening their crystalline deposits.

MINERALS—SOURCES AND EFFECTS

Great stories are also told about the special properties of minerals. Some of these claims probably arose to encourage children to eat their "greens"; others have their roots in generations of observation and folk wisdom. But whatever their origins, the table below will help you to unravel the truth.

MINERAL	SOURCES	SAID TO	ACTUALLY IS/DOES
CALCIUM	Dairy products, dried peas, canned sardines and salmon including bones, leafy green vegetables, oranges.	Build bones and teeth.	Build healthy bones and teeth. Regulate blood clotting and prevent muscle spasms.
CHROMIUM	Brewer's yeast, wheat germ, cheese.	Help hypoglycemia. Cure diabetes.	Important for glucose metabolism and insulin production, which are necessary for prevention of diabetes and hypoglycemia.
COPPER	Liver, kidneys, nuts, cocoa.	Cure anemia.	Necessary for the formation of red blood cells and absorption of iron.
FLUORIDE	Fluoridated water.	Cause cancer.	Contribute to strong bones and teeth.
IODINE	Seafood, eggs, iodized salt.	Cause anemia.	Keep skin, hair, and nails healthy. Maintain normal thyroid function. Prevent goiter.
IRON	Red meat, liver, eggs, dried beans, leafy green vegetables, molasses.	Control alcoholism and menstrual discomfort. Cure anemia.	Vital for the production of hemoglobin and myoglobin.
MAGNESIUM	Nuts, bananas, apricots, soybeans.	Cure heart disease. Help with alcoholism and prostate problems. Cure kidney stones.	Regulate heart rhythm. Needed for bone growth.
MANGANESE	Leafy green vegetables, tea.	Cure diabetes. Help fatigue and asthma. Cure sterility.	Necessary for normal cell function, bone growth, and reproduction.
POTASSIUM	Bananas, meats, potatoes, oranges, dried fruits.	Cure heart disease. Cure acne and arthritis. Alleviate alcoholism. Heal burns.	Regulate muscle contraction and blood pressure. Control water balance in tissues and cells.
PHOSPHORUS	Dairy products, meats, fish, nuts, whole grains, processed foods.	Cure arthritis. Accelerate children's growth. Reduce stress.	Promote strong teeth and bones. Necessary for energy metabolism.
SELENIUM	Seafood, garlic, tomatoes.	Cure cancer and arthritis.	Fight cell damage in conjunction with vitamin E.
SODIUM	Table salt, processed foods (for example, bacon, smoked fish).	Lower fever. Protect against cramping. Raise blood pressure.	Balance water in the body. Maintain high blood pressure.
ZINC	Oysters, meats, liver, wheat germ, pumpkin seeds, sunflower seeds.	Relieve angina and cirrhosis of the liver.	Important for normal growth, fetal growth, reproductive development, and the healing of wounds.

DEFICIENCIES

Various diseases were known for centuries before they were recognized as nutritional deficiencies that could be remedied through changes in diet.

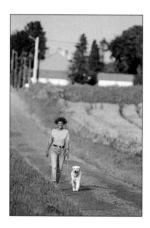

THE "SUNSHINE" VITAMIN
Sunshine is an important source of vitamin D. It is created when ultraviolet light in sunlight acts on a substance in the skin. People who remain indoors all day may become deficient in vitamin D, which can cause softened bones.

In 1746, James Lind proved that eating a lemon a day could prevent his sailors from developing scurvy, the potentially fatal disease that weakens the body's connective tissue. However, it took another 170 years before scientists isolated its cause—vitamin C deficiency. This important discovery soon led to uncovering the causes of a range of other deficiency diseases, including complete loss of eyesight (lack of vitamin A), beriberi, which is characterized by partial paralysis (lack of vitamin B_1), pellagra, which results in dermatitis, diarrhea, and dementia (lack of vitamin B_3), and rickets, a disease in which the bones do not harden properly and become distorted (lack of vitamin D). These diseases are now rare in the West, but the health of a fifth of the global population is damaged through a lack of adequate vitamins and minerals.

If you eat a varied diet that includes animal foods and plenty of fruits and vegetables, you will probably get all the vitamins and minerals you need. Certain groups of people, however, are still vulnerable to deficiencies. Vegetarians who eat no eggs, fish, or dairy products as well as no meat may not get enough B_{12}, causing new red blood cells to develop abnormally, without sufficient hemoglobin, necessary for carrying oxygen around the body. This condition is known as pernicious anemia. In spite of an increasing loss of sensation in the hands and feet, the disease may go unnoticed in children or the elderly until serious damage to the nervous system has already occurred.

People who stay indoors all day, such as institutionalized and very elderly people, may not get enough vitamin D. This may cause rickets in children and osteomalacia (softening of the bones) in adults.

Recommended dietary allowance

Different countries have established different recommended daily allowances (RDAs), the minimum amount of each vitamin and mineral needed to prevent deficiency (see pages 62-63). Levels in the United States are higher than they are in the United Kingdom, for instance, with a wider margin of nutritional safety. But RDAs tell you nothing about optimum requirements.

Many nutritionists are concerned that people do not eat a varied diet rich in fruits and vegetables (five servings per day) but instead one that contains too many snacks and fast foods. As a result, they believe that there is widespread inadequate nutrition—

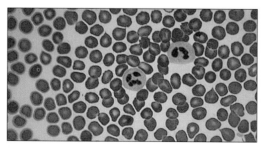

HEALTHY RED BLOOD CELLS
Red blood cells depend on iron, vitamin B_{12}, and folic acid to form hemoglobin, which transports oxygen to, and carbon dioxide from, the body's cells.

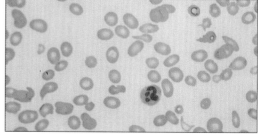

"SICK" RED BLOOD CELLS
A deficiency in vitamin B_{12} and folic acid can cause blood cells that lack hemoglobin and have less capacity for carrying oxygen; this gives rise to anemia.

many people with low or borderline levels of essential vitamins and minerals. Nutritionists are particularly worried about the levels of a range of minerals, including iron, calcium, zinc, magnesium, chromium, and selenium, and the vitamins A, C, and E.

IRON
Iron in red blood cells is efficiently recycled, and only a tiny amount is lost each day through feces, urine, and cells sloughed from the stomach. But even though iron is stored by the body, iron deficiency is the most common mineral deficiency worldwide. It occurs when the body does not get enough iron over a long period of time or because the body is lacking in other vital nutrients, such as B₆, folic acid, and magnesium. The body needs these nutrients in order to absorb iron.

In Western industrialized countries alone, it is estimated that as many as 20 to 30 percent of women of child-bearing age do not possess adequate iron reserves. In the United States, 4 to 10 percent of women in this age group are anemic. Inadequate intake, poor absorption, and blood loss through menstruation are the primary reasons for iron deficiency. Common symptoms are weakness, fatigue, and shortness of breath. According to the World Health Organization, about 700 million people

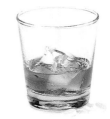

NUTRIENT DEPLETERS
Alcohol and some medications, such as antihistamines, diminish the beneficial effects of vitamin A.

CAUSES OF NUTRIENT DEPLETION

Vitamin loss occurs when foods are exposed to light and heat or are cooked in large amounts of water. After foods are eaten, the effects of their vitamins and minerals in the body diminishes if certain other substances are consumed.

NUTRIENT	BEFORE EATING	AFTER EATING
A	Light, air and iron or copper kitchen utensils.	An excess of alcohol, smoking, antihistamines, antacids.
B₁	Processing, heat, air, in alkaline conditions (cooked with baking soda), sulfur dioxide (preservative), leaching into cooking water.	An excess of alcohol, diuretics.
B₂	Light, heat, in alkaline conditions leaching into cooking water, milling of grains.	
B₃	Leaching into cooking water, milling of grains.	Isoniazid (antituberculous drug).
B₆	Freezing.	Excessive protein foods, diuretics.
B₁₂	Cooking, light, acidic conditions, oxidation.	An excess of alcohol, smoking.
FOLIC ACID	Processing at very high temperatures, light, leaching into cooking water.	An excess of alcohol, diuretics.
C	Prolonged warming, air, alkaline conditions, iron or copper kitchen utensils, leaching into water when soaked.	Smoking.
D	Alkaline conditions, light, air.	An excess of alcohol, antacids, laxatives, diuretics, anticonvulsive drugs.
E	Processing, light, heat, air, storing, alkali.	Polyunsaturated fats, laxatives.
K	Freezing, light, alkali.	Antibiotics, laxatives, diuretics.
CALCIUM AND ZINC	Not all minerals are destroyed by cooking or food preparation, but some leach into the cooking medium.	Smoking, caffeine, and diuretics affect calcium. Alcohol, caffeine, estrogen, diuretics, and antibiotics affect zinc.

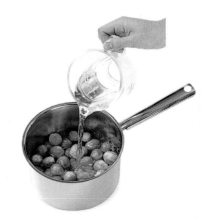

REDUCING LOSS OF NUTRIENTS
Boil vegetables in the minimum amount of water. Keep cooking time as short as possible.

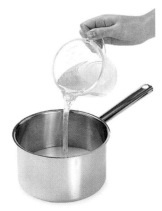

RECYCLING VITAMINS
Use the water that the vegetables were cooked in to make soups, sauces, or gravies.

worldwide have some degree of iron-deficiency anemia. Men and postmenopausal women usually have enough iron—their bodies store and recycle it efficiently. But the iron requirements of other groups may not be adequately met.

Women need extra iron during their fertile years. Menstruating women require more because of the monthly blood loss. Pregnant women need more iron because of increased blood volume and the requirements of the placenta and developing fetus.

Infants, children, and teenagers need more iron because of their rapid growth. Some studies have found that even minor iron deficiency may affect nonverbal learning and problem-solving capacity in children.

Dieters, especially women of child-bearing age, who eat only low-calorie meals are invariably getting an inadequate supply of iron and other nutrients to meet their needs.

Vegetarians, especially young vegetarian women, and people who eat little red meat should eat alternative iron-rich foods, such as dark green vegetables, fortified breakfast cereals, and apricots.

Getting enough iron

There are two forms of dietary iron: heme, derived from meat and meat products, and nonheme, which comes from vegetable sources. Iron absorption varies according to its source, with heme iron having a better rate of absorption than nonheme. On average, 25 percent of available heme iron is absorbed no matter what your body needs.

You can absorb a greater amount of both forms of iron by eating them with foods that are rich in vitamin C, such as cantaloupe, tomatoes, or cabbage. Foods that are calcium-rich, on the other hand, inhibit the body's ability to absorb iron. Also, the cooking method you choose can affect the iron content of the food. The heme iron in meat, for example, can be converted to nonheme iron if the meat is cooked for a long time at a high temperature.

CALCIUM

The bones act as a dynamic calcium storehouse for the rest of the body, continually losing and regaining calcium according to the body's needs. Hormones and vitamin D help to keep the calcium levels in the blood and other body fluids at a constant level, depositing any excess in the bones or removing it if needed elsewhere.

About 99 percent of the body's calcium is in the bones and teeth. The remaining 1 percent circulates in the blood, where it helps regulate muscle action, blood clotting, cell nourishment, release of energy, and transmission of nerve impulses. It may also play a role in helping to control blood pressure.

Peak bone mass

During growth, the skeleton increases in size, making extra demands on the body's calcium level. After growth stops, at about age 21 in boys and 18 in girls, the bone mass—the amount of bone and its calcium content together—continues to increase. At about age 30, what doctors term "peak bone mass" is achieved. (This depends on the degree to which the diet provided calcium and other related nutrients, such as vitamin D, zinc, copper, and manganese.) After this time, bone mass starts to decline very gradually because more bone is utilized by the body than is formed.

Because of hormonal changes, peak bone mass declines in a more pronounced manner in postmenopausal women. The decline in bone mass is normally not a problem for people whose calcium stores are adequate, but for those whose calcium intake was inadequate during the first three decades of life, the peak bone mass will not be enough to tolerate the gradual loss of bone mass over the years, and a deficiency condition, osteoporosis, will result (see opposite page).

Getting enough calcium

An inadequate calcium supply can occur if too little is consumed and absorbed or if too much is lost. Individuals at risk include growing infants, children, and adolescents; pregnant women, who lose it to the fetus; and nursing mothers, whose calcium-rich milk goes to the infant.

Also at risk are postmenopausal women, at least half of whom suffer loss of bone density, and people who smoke and/or consume excessive amounts of alcohol, caffeinated beverages, and high-protein foods such as meat, all of which increase the rate at which calcium is excreted.

The United States has set a Recommended Daily Allowance (RDA) of 1,200 milligrams of calcium for people between the ages of 11 and 25. The allowance is high because this age group has the most efficient calcium absorption and can store it for later years.

PREGNANCY
Lack of folic acid is linked with an increased risk of having a baby with a defect such as spina bifida. Pregnant women, therefore, need to eat more foods that contain folic acid, such as spinach. Moreover, women who are hoping to become pregnant are advised to take supplements because the defect occurs in the 26th to 28th day of development, before most women know they are pregnant.

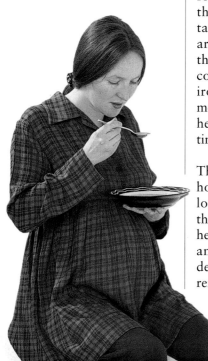

VITAMIN AND MINERAL SUPPLEMENTS

A huge profit is made by the companies and pundits who market vitamin and mineral supplements—around one in three adults takes the supplements regularly. However, it is still not known how much good such supplements do for people who ordinarily are in good health.

A balanced diet that includes a variety of fresh fruit and vegetables will probably supply you with all the vitamins and minerals that you will need. However, many factors can impair the nutritional content of these normally healthful foods. The amount of time it takes to transport fruits and vegetables to the place of purchase, whether they were stored before shipping and for how long, and whether or not the produce is seasonal will greatly affect its nutritional value. Certain vitamins, most notably C, degrade very quickly, and the vitamin C content of foods such as of apples, broccoli, and strawberries has been found to vary widely.

Preparation and cooking, especially cooking with high heat and lots of water, also affect nutritional content; the retention of many vitamins can be as little as 40 percent of the original values.

In addition, many people just eat unwisely, and everyone has days when there is only time for snacks. Moreover, certain groups of people have higher than average nutritional requirements—people who are ill, the elderly, heavy drinkers and smokers, strict vegetarians and vegans, crash dieters and fussy eaters, athletes, children, and pregnant and breast-feeding women. For those people with inadequate dietary intakes, a nutritional boost provided by fortified meal replacements, such as breakfast cereals, or a supplement may be worthwhile.

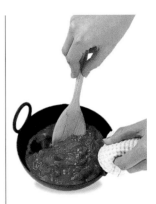

COOKING TO ADD IRON
You can improve the iron content of certain foods by cooking them in an iron pot or pan. Acidic foods, such as tomatoes, leach iron from the pot, which then becomes available as dietary iron.

THE EFFECTS OF OSTEOPOROSIS

Calcium is essential for bone health; without it, bones become brittle and weak and prone to fracture. This condition is called osteoporosis, and it affects women much more than men.

Estrogen, a hormone vital for the metabolism of calcium, is produced by both men and women. A woman's main source, however, comes from her ovaries, and after menopause, they stop producing it. At that time calcium is incorporated into bone less efficiently and is also lost at a faster rate. The result is a bone structure that becomes progressively weaker. Osteoporosis becomes even more likely if a woman had poor bone density early in life, smokes, or eats a low-calcium diet.

Many gynecologists recommend hormone replacement therapy (HRT) for women who are at risk of osteoporosis, as well as eating calcium-rich foods like dark leafy greens and yogurt. The 1994 National Institutes of Health Consensus Conference suggested that women over 40 who are not on HRT take the equivalent of 1,500 milligrams of calcium a day, and that women over 40 on HRT take at least 1,000 milligrams. Small amounts of zinc, copper, and manganese enhance the absorption of calcium.

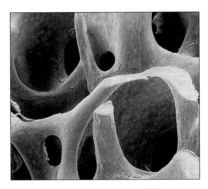

HEALTHY BONE
Calcium-rich bone maintains a resilient internal structure. This keeps it resistant to fracture. Eating foods rich in calcium and regularly doing impact exercise, such as walking, help to keep bones strong.

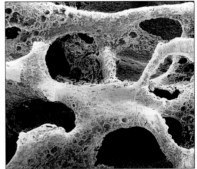

OSTEOPOROTIC BONE
Bone tissue affected by osteoporosis is much less dense, more brittle, and prone to fracture. Your diet and the amount of weight-bearing exercise you did in your twenties and early thirties influence your chance of developing the condition.

HIP FRACTURE RISKS
After the age of 50, there is an increasing risk of osteoporotic hip fracture. Naturally occurring low levels of estrogen, combined with insufficient calcium intake, make the possibility of bone fractures more likely.

Cumulative risk, %

40
30
20
10
0

Age 55 60 65 70 75 80 85 90

Females   Males

How to buy and take supplements

Nutrient supplements may consist of a single micronutrient, such as vitamin C or iron, or be combinations of vitamins and minerals. The latter are generally more expensive and are available in a wide range of combinations and dosages.

Always buy from a store with a high turnover and check the "sell by" date on the container.

Store vitamins and minerals in a cool, dry place—where you will not forget to take them—but make sure that they are not within reach of children.

Take supplements according to the manufacturer's recommendations. In general, they should be taken with or immediately after food. On an empty stomach they are less efficient because their major role is to aid the metabolism of protein, fat, and carbohydrates.

Overdosing on supplements

Many people consume large quantities of certain supplements, especially vitamin C and iron, in the belief that a high amount will increase the beneficial effects. However, megadoses—an amount that is 10 times or more than the RDA—can be harmful.

The vitamins A, D, and E are stored in fat and can build up in the body. If taken regularly, doses of vitamins A and D that are 5 to 10 times higher than the RDA can be toxic. People have become very ill from eating large quantities of animal liver, which contains a great deal of vitamin A. Fish liver oil is a rich source of both A and D, but if you have too much, you are likely to vomit.

There does not appear to be any danger from a prolonged high intake of beta carotene. The only side effect is a yellowing of the skin, particularly the palms of the hands and soles of the feet. But recent studies have shown there is no benefit from megadoses.

Vitamin E is not toxic in high doses either. One hundred milligrams a day appears to be beneficial in thwarting heart disease, but some people take larger doses because they

SYMPTOMS OF NUTRIENT DEFICIENCY

Everybody needs a balanced intake of vitamins and minerals. Some people, however, require a greater intake to meet particular needs. If they do not get an adequate supply, these people may suffer problems that are signs of the nutrient deficiency.

NUTRIENT	DEFICIENCY SYMPTOMS	THOSE MOST AT RISK
A	Dry eyes, night blindness, poor growth and development, hardening of skin, impaired immunity.	Toddlers.
B$_1$	Fatigue, muscle weakness, and nausea. Can lead to fatal illness called beriberi with heart failure.	Alcoholics, people on a subsistence diet of polished rice.
B$_2$	Dry and cracked skin, bloodshot eyes, sore lips and tongue.	People who do not drink milk.
B$_3$	Depression and tiredness. Severe deficiency leads to pellagra, which is characterized by dermatitis, diarrhea, and dementia.	People on a corn-based diet.
B$_6$	Convulsions.	Naturally occurring deficiency unknown.
B$_{12}$	Megaloblastic anemia (abnormal red blood cells). Degeneration of the spinal cord, which leads to paralysis and death. May also cause mental confusion in the elderly.	Vegetarians (especially vegans), heavy drinkers, pregnant and lactating women. Deficiency usually caused by malabsorption rather than dietary lack.
C	Slow wound healing, loose teeth, bleeding gums, easy bruising, recurrent infections, internal hemorrhaging, scurvy.	Smokers, the elderly.
D	Rickets (bones do not harden and become distorted in children), osteomalacia (softening of the bones in adults).	Children, the elderly, the housebound, individuals consuming a diet rich in unleavened bread and brown rice.
E	Hemolytic anemia, nerve damage.	Individuals with a diet low in polyunsaturated fats, especially fish oils.
CALCIUM	Rickets, osteomalacia.	Children, adolescents, pregnant and lactating women, vegans, the elderly.
IRON	Iron-deficiency anemia—fatigue, shortness of breath.	Women who have heavy periods, pregnant women, vegetarians, sick or elderly people.

believe doing so will prolong life. However, the long-term effects of continuing high doses of vitamin E are not known.

Vitamin C and the B family, which are water soluble, are not stored in the body, and so do not build to toxic levels. Still, excesses can precipitate problems. Megadoses of B_3 can cause nausea, flushing, and low blood pressure. Too much B_6, which some women take for premenstrual syndrome, can lead to irreversible nerve damage. Avoid doses exceeding 25 milligrams per day. An excess of folic acid can mask symptoms of pernicious anemia, making it difficult to diagnose. Sudden high doses of vitamin C may cause gastric disturbances.

Ideally, you should take supplements only on the recommendation of your doctor. Tests can establish whether or not a supplement is needed, especially when you are thinking of taking iron, selenium, or zinc. Each can build up in toxic amounts that may damage body tissues or organs, including the liver, pancreas, and heart.

No mineral should be routinely consumed in doses greater than 10 times the RDA, and even that practice should be short term.

Can disease be treated with vitamins?

The most publicized claims for the use of a vitamin in the treatment of disease are those of the American scientist, Linus Pauling (1901–94). Initially, he advocated the use of gram doses of vitamin C to ward off and treat colds, but later he went further, suggesting that vitamin C could prevent all manner of human diseases, even cancer.

Pauling's unorthodox methods and sweeping claims eventually earned him the suspicion of the medical and scientific communities. Many studies were conducted to test his idea that vitamin C was a cold curative, but most of them indicated only small

continued on page 74

TREATING DISEASE

In some cases, vitamin and mineral supplements move out of the realm of preventive medicine and into that of treatment. Doctors have discovered that many diseases and conditions can be relieved with proper supplementation. All these applications should be under the supervision of a doctor or clinical nutritionist.

▶ *Fat-soluble vitamins A, D, E, and K can help people with cystic fibrosis, pancreatic diseases, and malabsorption problems.*

▶ *Vitamin B_{12} (by injection) aids people who have had an operation on the stomach or small intestine. It is also given to people who have difficulty metabolizing vitamin B_{12}.*

▶ *Vitamin B_3 (niacin) lowers blood cholesterol.*

▶ *Vitamin B_6 eases premenstrual tension.*

▶ *All B vitamins are recommended for individuals with alcoholism, because they help to heal the damage caused by excess alcohol consumption.*

▶ *Chromium helps to correct glucose intolerance.*

PREVENTING DISEASE WITH FOOD

Evidence from over 300 studies has suggested that people who eat large quantities of the foods containing antioxidants—vitamins E, C, and beta carotene—have a reduced risk of many cancers, heart disease, cataracts, and stroke. Vitamin D also has disease-preventing properties, helping to stave off osteoporosis. It is the food itself that is particularly valuable, not the isolated nutrient that is found in supplements. Fruits and vegetables contain natural substances that enhance the absorption of vitamins and perhaps provide protection from disease.

SOURCES OF BETA CAROTENE
Orange, red, and yellow vegetables and fruits are high in beta carotene and other carotenes that may help to reduce the risk of lung cancer. The fiber in these foods may contribute to a reduced risk of colon cancer.

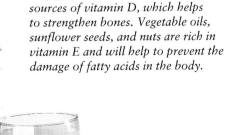

SOURCES OF VITAMINS D AND E
Oily fish and fortified milks are good sources of vitamin D, which helps to strengthen bones. Vegetable oils, sunflower seeds, and nuts are rich in vitamin E and will help to prevent the damage of fatty acids in the body.

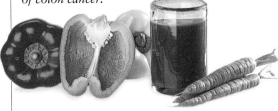

SOURCES OF VITAMIN C
Citrus fruits, broccoli, and potatoes are rich in vitamin C, which is an effective cancer preventer and helps to block the formation of cancer-causing nitrosamines.

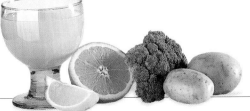

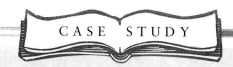
A Perimenopausal Woman

The time leading up to menopause can be very challenging—the body you thought you knew undergoes a major internal transformation. As hormones ebb and flow, emotional changes, like moodiness and irritability, and physical ones, such as hot flashes and joint pain, may arise. You can help to counteract these effects by making positive changes in your diet, exercise patterns, and attitude.

Ellen is a 47-year-old single executive. She recently left her job in a public relations firm to start her own business. Since then she has done hardly anything else but work. She has stopped seeing friends and exercising and no longer pays much attention to what she eats.

She starts her day with four cups of coffee, then snacks on cookies, chocolate, potato chips, and similar fare until dinner. Then she usually grabs a bowl of pasta, washed down with a glass or two of wine to help her to unwind. Despite her poor eating habits and lack of exercise, she does not have a weight problem and has felt great, until recently. Now she is constantly tired, as well as short-tempered and irritable.

Ellen's menstrual cycle has also become irregular. In addition, she is sweating a lot. At first, she broke out into a sweat every afternoon, but now it happens twice a day. She feels frustrated by her lack of control over her own body and blames the stress of her business for her symptoms.

Frightened by her feelings of powerlessness, Ellen took a two-week holiday. As she unwound from the pressures of her job, she thought about what was happening to her. Could it be menopause? She is sure this happens later and thinks her symptoms are simply stress related.

Once back at work, she resumes her usual frenetic pace and finds that her symptoms have escalated. To keep her energy level up, she drinks more coffee and eats more sugary snacks. At night, to wind down, she drinks an extra glass of wine. But she finds that no matter how much sugar and caffeine she consumes, she still lacks energy. In addition, her nightly drinks no longer relax her. Ellen decides she needs to get help.

DIET
Sufficient calcium intake is essential as a woman ages, to replace that being lost from the body. Eating a balanced diet (see page 18) will also improve mood and attitude, as well as relieve many menopausal symptoms.

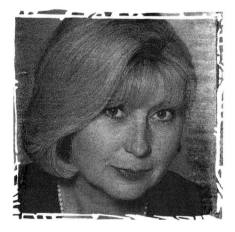

HEALTH
Physical symptoms, such as hot flashes, night sweats, aches in the joints, and stress incontinence, are a few of the conditions associated with the onset of the menopause. Hot flashes can last for just a few seconds or up to several minutes.

FITNESS
A lack of exercise can exacerbate the emotional symptoms of menopause, such as anxiety and depression. Inactivity can also increase the risks of osteoporosis and heart disease.

EATING HABITS
A busy and active life tends to leave little time for specially prepared and relaxed meals. Taking time to prepare meals will relieve tension.

EMOTIONAL HEALTH
Around the time of menopause, women may experience disconcerting mood swings. Anxiety and tearfulness can arise with only slight provocation and be followed by sudden inexplicable euphoria.

WHAT SHOULD ELLEN DO?

Rather than reaching for coffee, sugar, and alcohol, Ellen needs to take an honest look at what is going on in her life. Although her stress level has not really changed much, she seems less able to cope with it.

Ellen should make an appointment with her general practitioner or gynecologist to find out whether she is undergoing menopause. Menopause has a number of serious health implications—notably increased risks of osteoporosis (see page 69) and heart disease.

To find out more about what is happening to her body, Ellen should read more about female health. There are many books about women's health and menopause in bookstores, and her local public library may also have a selection of relevant literature. Ellen could also talk to friends who have already experienced menopause.

In addition, Ellen could become more familiar with the different therapies that may help to relieve menopausal symptoms. Hormone replacement therapy (HRT) works well to relieve hot flashes and night sweats and helps to avert osteoporosis and heart disease.

Relaxation therapies such as meditation can also offer relief, as they calm the mind and body.

All this information will help to make Ellen feel more in control of what is going on in her body.

Action Plan

DIET
Find out about the diet recommended for women going through menopause. (High-calcium foods, such as dairy products, are important for staving off osteoporosis.) Ellen also needs a good intake of vitamin D to aid the absorption and metabolism of calcium. Caffeine is a calcium depleter.

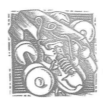

FITNESS
Plan to exercise regularly—at least three times a week. Brisk walking, aerobics, and walking on a treadmill help to strengthen bone mass, which reduces the risk of osteoporosis. Decide whether to take up a sport or join a fitness club.

HEALTH
Arrange to see a doctor. (May need various health checks—pelvic and breast examinations, including a mammogram and cervical smear—as well as height, weight, blood pressure, and cholesterol. Have hormone levels measured through a blood test.) Self-examine breasts once a month.

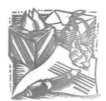

EMOTIONAL HEALTH
Contact a local self-help group. Learn to anticipate mood swings and investigate various natural and medical remedies. For example, certain herbal preparations are said to be calming. HRT is effective for emotional symptoms and helps to increase energy levels.

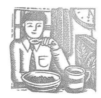

EATING HABITS
Take time to prepare meals. If too busy or tired during the week, make more time-consuming, nourishing meals on the weekend and freeze uneaten food in portion-size containers. Reheat the food after work or the gym. Stop snacking on chocolates and cookies. Try eating smaller meals frequently.

HOW THINGS TURN OUT FOR ELLEN

Ellen's gynecologist tells her she is perimenopausal. This stage, which may last several years, precedes the last menstrual period. Hormone levels begin to drop, and during this time many physical symptoms of menopause, such as hot flashes and night sweats, are experienced. Ellen's doctor recommends a nutritionist, who provides a diet to help Ellen's body cope with its changes. This new diet consists of four well-balanced low-fat, high-fiber meals a day. She has to eat plenty of whole grains, fresh fruits and vegetables, and small amounts of fish and lean meats.

Ellen now drinks only one cup of coffee a day and has cut down on fast food. She also drinks more water to replace the amount she loses through sweating. For snacks she eats calcium-rich foods like low-fat milk, yogurt, and cheese. Eating regular, nutritious meals gives her more energy and reduces her moodiness and irritability.

In the evening Ellen stops work an hour early and walks part of the way home. She has joined a health club with a friend, and several days a week she spends some time exercising at the gym or at home. She has gotten much better at unwinding, and the combination of exercise and relaxation is invigorating.

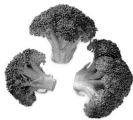

VITAMIN C
Just 3½ oz of broccoli supply more than double the Recommended Daily Allowance for vitamin C.

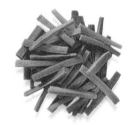

BETA CAROTENE
Eating a 1¼-oz carrot meets the daily need for beta carotene.

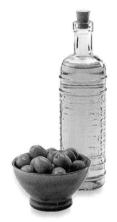

VITAMIN E
Vegetable oils are a good source of vitamin E. Use unsaturated oils— for example, olive—when cooking instead of the more harmful saturated fats, such as butter.

positive effects in reducing the incidence, easing the symptoms, and shortening the duration of the common cold.

Recently, however, interest in vitamin C as a possible means of preventing colds has revived. Recognition of vitamin C's antioxidant properties and its enhancement of immune functions has led to more research, and some of Pauling's initial observations are stimulating further investigation as well.

FREE RADICALS AND ANTIOXIDANTS

Research has uncovered so-called unstable molecules (free radicals), which may be causal factors in a number of degenerative diseases, including cancer and heart disease. This theory has led to further investigations to clarify the relationship between free radical molecules and antioxidants, such as beta carotene, which mop them up and may therefore reduce the risk of these diseases. Several studies suggest that vitamin A and possibly the other carotenes may help to prevent breast cancer.

The evidence that vitamin E reduces the incidence of heart disease is even stronger. In one European study, 16,000 men between 40 and 59 years of age from 16 different places were tested. The higher the level of vitamin E in their blood, the lower their death rates from heart disease. Similar associations have been observed for vitamin C and beta carotene. All are antioxidants, and it appears that they function as a protective "brigade" with vitamin C as the first line of defense, vitamin E and other compounds in the middle, and beta carotene as a last line of defense against free radicals.

However, these findings do not mean that you should start taking supplements of these antioxidants. Although the effects of vitamin supplements are still being debated, there is no question that eating more fruit, vegetables, and grains rich in antioxidants is beneficial. It is therefore advisable to make sure you follow the current dietary recommendations for these foods. To ensure an adequate intake of vitamins, minerals, and other nutrients, health experts recommend that you consume a certain number of food portions each day: 6 to 11 servings of bread, cereals, pasta, and rice; 5 servings of fruits and vegetables; 2 to 3 servings of dairy products, preferably low-fat or nonfat; 2 to 3 servings of protein foods, such as meat, seafood, legumes, and eggs; and only a very small amount of fat.

ALUMINUM AND ALZHEIMER'S DISEASE

Alzheimer's disease is a condition—to date irreversible—in which the brain's nerve cells progressively degenerate and cause the brain to shrink. In different studies scientists have found high levels of aluminum in the brain of some Alzheimer's patients and a concentration of cases in areas with high concentrations of aluminum in the drinking water.

But controversy rages about whether excessive aluminum is the cause, or a result, of the neurological damage in Alzheimer's disease. Scientists are not sure that changes in the brain and other organs in the body are caused by the disease. Alzheimer's might ease the entry of aluminum and other metals to the brain.

However, in the wake of the evidence linking Alzheimer's and aluminum, many people have become concerned over the safety of aluminum cooking utensils. But even if the metal does leach into food,

scientists are not sure if dietary aluminum can be absorbed through the intestines. It is now thought that drinking plenty of fluids and eating a balanced diet may be of more practical benefit in warding off Alzheimer's disease than attempting to be sure that no aluminum enters your diet through cooking utensils. You can, however, choose from a wide range of pots and pans made in other materials, particularly stainless steel and ceramic.

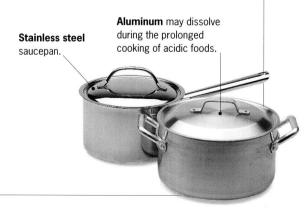

Stainless steel saucepan.

Aluminum may dissolve during the prolonged cooking of acidic foods.

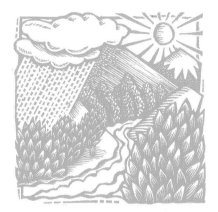

CHAPTER 6

THE FLUID FACTOR

*What you drink and when and how much
is as important to a healthy diet as the food
you eat. All living cells and organs need water to
function. Water is the basis of essential body
fluids such as blood and lymph, it lubricates joints,
it is needed to form saliva, it provides a protective
cushion for the body's tissues, and it helps to
eliminate digestive waste from the body. Water,
skim milk, and unsweetened fruit juices are the
most beneficial fluids, while alcoholic and
caffeine-filled drinks—tea, coffee, and certain
colas—may be harmful if taken in excess.*

ARE YOU DRINKING ENOUGH WATER?

You can live for several weeks without food, but without water you will die in just a few days. Most North Americans have a ready source, although there may be doubts about its quality.

THE RIGHT AMOUNT

As a rough guide, the World Health Organization recommends that everyone drink eight 8-ounce glasses of water a day. Drink more water if

▶ *You take part in strenuous exercise.*

▶ *The weather is hot.*

▶ *You are at a high altitude.*

▶ *You are ill, especially with diarrhea or fever.*

▶ *You are menopausal and suffering from hot flashes and night sweats.*

In 1987 the people of Greece endured a 10-day heat wave during which temperatures reached 110°F. More than 1,000 inhabitants died, most of them elderly, mainly from dehydration—loss of fluids and body salt. This is an extreme example of what can happen if the body is not kept properly hydrated. Clearly, the high temperature was the major contributing factor in the tragedy, but even in moderate temperatures, it is important to drink enough water to replace the amount lost through bodily functions—breathing, perspiration, urination, and defecation.

On average, you lose two to four pints of water a day. This rate will increase significantly, up to as much as nine pints, through perspiration during periods of heavy physical exertion or very hot weather, also at high elevations. As long as the lost fluid is replenished, there is no problem. But other factors, such as an ill state of health, can lead to a dangerous increase in water loss. Fever, vomiting, diarrhea, and blood loss all cause dehydration. Treatment for these illnesses includes the controlled replacement of lost water.

AN ADEQUATE SUPPLY

If the body does not take in enough water, those functions requiring the action of water, such as the dilution and evacuation of toxins, lead to water being drawn from the cells to make up the balance. This results in dehydration of the cells, which shrivel and cease to function properly. The body reacts swiftly to water loss: losing just 1 percent is enough to make us thirsty, while extreme rates of dehydration can lead to heat exhaustion and may even be fatal.

SUFFERING FROM THE EFFECTS OF HEAT

Insufficient water intake is one of the main causes of heat exhaustion—signaled by cramps, nausea, and headache. Sufferers will also have shallow breathing and clammy skin. If heat exhaustion is not treated, heatstroke may develop: sweating stops, the skin becomes flushed, and there may be loss of consciousness, coma, and death. An individual suffering from heat exhaustion should lie in a cool place and sip an oral rehydration solution—1 teaspoon of salt and 8 teaspoons of sugar in 3½ cups of water. If he becomes unconscious, place him in a prone position with the head facing right or left until consciousness is regained. Then administer the rehydration solution. Seek medical help immediately.

HEAT EXHAUSTION
A sufferer will feel nauseated and sweat profusely. The diagram below shows the response of skin to heat.

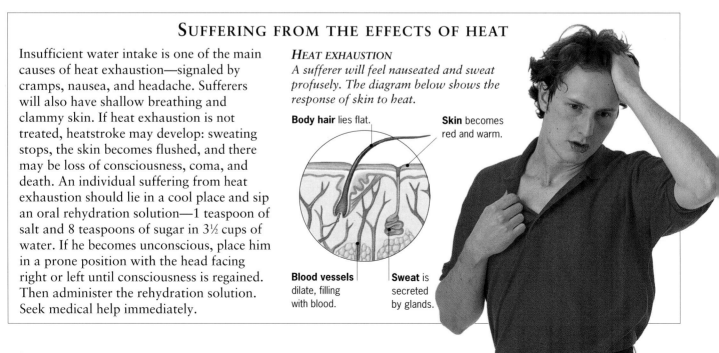

Body hair lies flat.

Skin becomes red and warm.

Blood vessels dilate, filling with blood.

Sweat is secreted by glands.

Dehydration becomes a major threat when 10 percent of a person's weight is lost.

The sensation of thirst is the body's way of saying that it needs more water. A dry mouth is the result of the blood becoming excessively salty and drawing moisture from the salivary glands to redress the balance. Usually a glass or two of water is enough to stop you from feeling thirsty, but it may not be enough to prevent dehydration.

Thirst is an imperfect warning system, however, because it is not triggered until dehydration has already begun. Therefore your thirst may tend to be quenched before you have drunk an adequate amount of water. So it is a good idea to drink enough water to satisfy the thirst and then drink some more—another glass or two. If you are constantly thirsty, however, see your doctor. Excessive thirst can also be a sign of diabetes mellitus.

Are you drinking the right water?

Water from the tap in most developed countries has long been taken for granted as safe to drink. In recent years, however, many people have become concerned about pollutants seeping into the water supply, and the rising sales of filters and bottled water reflect this general unease.

Tap water comes from two main sources: surface water and groundwater. Surface water includes lakes, reservoirs, rivers, and streams, which supply most major cities, while groundwater—a more common source for rural areas—comes from underground sources, such as springs and aquifers where water collects.

The treatment of water

With their several stages of filtration, aeration, and disinfection, modern water-treatment systems are highly sophisticated, and most of the water supplied to the public is safe to drink. This is particularly true for urban areas where the consumer is served by municipal water systems. In rural areas, where the demand on small community systems is greater, and especially where water is drawn from private wells, extra vigilance is more important.

The risk of becoming ill as a result of consuming contaminated drinking water is very small. Most drinking water is safer now than it has ever been. This statement is borne out by the low incidence of disease

WATERY FOODS

Half the water your body needs comes from foods. Vegetables and fruits contain more liquid than solid matter.

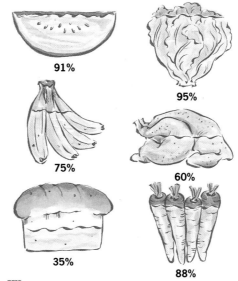

91%

95%

75%

60%

35%

88%

WATER LEVELS IN FOOD
Watermelons are almost entirely water, while the proportion of water in lettuce is 95 percent, in carrots 88 percent, and in bananas about 75 percent. Poultry is about 60 percent water, and water even makes up about 35 percent of bread.

WHICH DRINK IS BEST?

Almost any fluid will do for replenishment, but water, pure and simple, is best. The next best are pure fruit juices and low-fat or nonfat milk. Caffeine and alcoholic drinks do not replace lost water because they act as diuretics, making the kidneys produce more urine than they would normally. Drinking sweet carbonated drinks increases the amount of sugar in your diet, which may cause tooth decay.

QUENCHING
YOUR THIRST
Choose plain water, juice, or skim milk instead of alcoholic, caffeinated, or carbonated drinks.

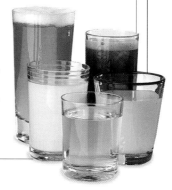

Fluid intake and exercise

During periods of prolonged strenuous exercise, such as cycling or marathon running, it is particularly important to replenish the extra fluid that is lost. Many nutritionists recommend that endurance athletes take sports drinks to rehydrate the body. These commercial drinks contain small amounts of carbohydrates and sodium and are absorbed by the body faster than water. The carbohydrates also supply needed fuel.

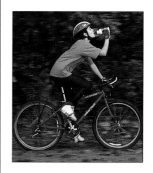

REPLENISHING FLUIDS
While exercising, have a sports drink or a glass of water every 15 to 20 minutes.

Filtering water

Water filters are an inexpensive and popular way of cleaning water. Some filters consist of layers of activated charcoal (charcoal that is honeycombed with tiny channels). As water passes through these channels, chemicals and some metals stick to the walls and are filtered out. But if the activated charcoal or carbon filters are not changed regularly, they can become a breeding ground for harmful bacteria. Also, charcoal filters generally do not eliminate lead and other heavy metals or nitrates. However, there are types of filter cartridges available for lead removal. The best approach for treating water is to have it tested and then consult an expert for the best solution.

caused by contaminated water today compared to the time before chlorination and controls on water sourcing were imposed. But the quantity of chemicals and metals being discharged into the environment by industrial plants and modern agricultural methods is putting a burden on water sources, and inevitably some pollution will occur. Unfortunately, the appearance, taste, and smell of the water you drink are not effective criteria for determining its quality. Many pollutants do not make water look or taste different.

In the United States water companies are required to conduct stringent tests in order to comply with Environmental Protection Agency regulations. This agency's standards are among the highest in the world, so public water supplies are generally safe. If you are worried about the quality of your water supply, contact your local company, which will provide details on their water-quality records or visit your home and test your water. If you have well water, you must take responsibility for having samples of it tested.

Bacterial and organic pollutants

Whether natural or synthetic, organic chemicals are usually found in very dilute amounts in drinking water. There is therefore no clear evidence of a link to health problems. However, despite the improvements brought about by disinfection of water supplies, disease-causing microbes in drinking water have caused some concern. In groundwater areas the source can be leaking septic tanks or animal feedlot wastes, while surface water supplies can be affected by inadequate treatment of water from poorly maintained purification plants.

A common test for water purity is to monitor for the presence of coliform bacteria. Often harmless themselves, they indicate the presence of other disease-causing microbes. An average count of one or more coliforms per 100 milliliters of water is enough to require an area of coastal water to be declared unsuitable for bathing.

Contamination by organic chemicals is not new. Most of the chemicals are formed from decaying matter and therefore occur naturally. In addition to these pollutants, there are numerous synthetic organic chemicals developed in industrial solvents, pesticides, and herbicides.

Chlorination

Very occasionally chlorination itself, used to cleanse water of infectious organisms, can create cancer-causing substances, such as chloroform, from organic matter found in the water supply. The risk is slight, however, and the benefits vastly outweigh the possible disadvantages.

THREATS TO THE WATER SUPPLY

A range of pollutants can enter a surface water supply through acid rain, pesticide runoff in rural and suburban areas, rainwater runoff in cities, and industrial waste from manufacturing plants. Groundwater supplies are exposed to a more limited range of pollutants, but generally in higher concentrations. Fertilizers sink down through the soil, and chemical wastes seep from poorly maintained sunken fuel tanks, waste-storage sites, or simply from carelessly discarded household products.

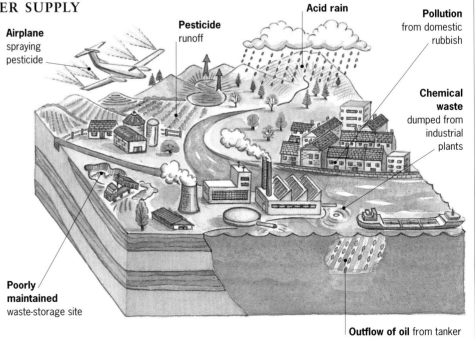

Airplane spraying pesticide

Pesticide runoff

Acid rain

Pollution from domestic rubbish

Chemical waste dumped from industrial plants

Poorly maintained waste-storage site

Outflow of oil from tanker

REDUCING LEAD

If you live in an area where the water is soft, you can carry out a basic filtering measure for lead by following these simple steps.

▶ *Do not use hot water for drinking or cooking, since hot water dissolves more lead from pipes.*

▶ *Let your tap run cold for a while first thing in the morning. Lead can build up overnight or in water that has sat in the pipe for a few hours. Flushing the toilet or running the shower will also help to wash the pipes of any accumulated levels of lead.*

▶ *Let water run for a few seconds before drinking from the cold tap during the day.*

Heavy metals

People living in a chalk or limestone area have hard water, which contains calcium salts that make the water slightly alkaline. Those who live in a granite area have soft water, which is fairly acidic. Lead, copper, and cadmium seep into the water supply in areas where the water is soft because soft water has a more corrosive effect on the metals used in water pipes than hard water.

Of all the heavy metals, the most dangerous is probably lead because of its high toxicity, menacing the developing brain and nervous systems of fetuses and children. Lead is usually not present in water sources but gets into drinking water because of the action of soft water on lead pipes, which were once used to connect properties to the water main and for solder in household plumbing. Lead has not been used for these purposes since the late 1970's, but some older homes still have lead in their systems. If you think your household is at risk, ask your water company to test your water.

The question of fluoride

Fluoride is an essential micronutrient that is used to strengthen teeth (particularly children's) by forming mineral crystals in the tooth enamel. Fluoride both strengthens the enamel and prevents naturally occurring bacteria from causing decay. Most doctors believe that fluoride is quite safe, yet some claim that it can be dangerous. They point to a few studies that have linked it to increased incidence of cancer, reduced thyroid activity, and erosion of the stomach

lining. The methodology of these studies has been questioned, however, and most scientists discount them. Communities in which the water is fluoridated have shown no increase in the incidence of cancer or any other of the alleged ill effects.

At one part per million parts of water—the standard level of flouride used in water fluoridation—fluoride is perfectly safe, and helps to reduce the risk of dental caries. The only adverse effect is found in regions with water supplies that have naturally occurring high levels of fluoride (about eight times the level used in artificially fluoridated supplies). In these areas there have been cases of dental fluorosis, a pitting and discoloration of the teeth. Children who still have their first set of teeth are particularly at risk from fluorosis, and should brush their teeth with toothpastes containing the lowest levels of fluoride. Most brands of toothpaste, however, are safe for use by the whole family.

IS MINERAL WATER MORE HEALTHFUL THAN TAP WATER?

Bottled mineral water, both still and sparkling, was one of the growth industries of the last decade. The minerals most often found in mineral water are calcium, magnesium, potassium, and sulfate. Many claims are made about the health benefits of mineral waters, but although some may taste better, they are unlikely to have much effect on health one way or the other. In addition, the sudden boom in mineral water sales means that regulation has yet to keep pace fully, and both the levels of purity and the claims made about beneficial effects are open to doubt. The high mineral content of some waters makes them unsuitable for babies and young children, while people with high blood pressure should avoid waters with a high sodium content. Check the labels of the various brands.

While there is no hard and fast evidence that mineral water provides greater safety than tap water, it can be a useful, if often expensive, alternative in the event of short-term pollution. In general, bottled water should always be drunk in countries where the purity of the water supply is questionable—and in such places it should also used for brushing your teeth. But where water conditions are deemed acceptable, bottled water does not usually provide any greater level of safety.

Rocketing sales
The amount of bottled water consumed has been rising for more than a decade. In the United States, sales have increased from 3.6 billion liters in 1982 to 8.5 billion liters in 1992. Whether for health, fashion, or preference, the market is growing increasingly larger each year.

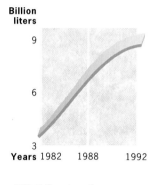

Billion liters

U.S. sales of bottled water

Drinking mineral water in restaurants
If you are concerned about the purity of water in a restaurant, order bottled water and make sure the bottle is opened in front of you so that you know the original contents have not been replaced by water from the tap or from a soda siphon.

To your health

Intrigued by an unexpectedly low rate of heart disease in France, researchers looked at the French diet and discovered that substances in red wine may hold the key to a healthy heart.

SENSIBLE DRINKING

Drinking alcohol may help you to relax, but too much can affect your nervous system. To remain in control, follow these tips.

Do

▶ *Sip your drinks slowly and develop the habit of putting your glass down between sips.*

▶ *Drink water and wine alternately.*

▶ *Know your limit and stick to it.*

▶ *Give yourself two alcohol-free days per week.*

Don't

▶ *Become involved in drinking "rounds."*

▶ *Mix your drinks.*

▶ *Drink alcohol to quench a thirst. Use water for that.*

▶ *Instinctively refill your glass when it is empty.*

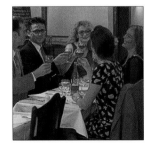

STAYING IN CONTROL Make sure you have something to eat before you have a drink and while you drink.

The French are justly famed for their food and wines, so their high-cholesterol diet—cassoulet, croissants, pâté de foie gras—and their reputation as Europe's major smokers and wine drinkers, along with their lukewarm attitude toward exercise, would seem to be a recipe for rampant heart disease. Yet the incidence of heart disease in France is far lower than in the rest of Europe or North America.

French adults drink an average of 2.5 glasses of red wine a day and often let their children drink watered-down wine at mealtimes. In recent years some scientists have put forward the theory that this habit of drinking red wine may indeed help to prevent heart disease.

PROTECTING YOUR HEART

Alcohol raises the levels of protective substances in the blood called high-density lipoproteins (HDLs), which actively remove cholesterol. The less cholesterol there is in the blood, the less chance there is of the arteries clogging up with fatty deposits and bringing on a heart attack.

All alcohol, drunk in moderation, has this effect, but naturally occurring tannins and other chemicals in red wine are thought to slow the oxidation of dietary lipids, keeping them active longer.

A healthy amount

The operative term is "moderate." Experts emphasize that the window of opportunity for deriving positive effects from alcohol is quite narrow—up to two drinks a day for men and no more than one for women. Otherwise, the bad effects start to outweigh the good. A "drink" here means 4 fluid ounces of wine or 16 ounces of beer.

Moderate consumption of red wine also reduces the stickiness of blood platelets, helping to prevent blood clots. As all alcohol produces this effect, people with bleeding conditions, such as hemophilia, should avoid drinking alcohol because it can bring on cerebral hemorrhaging.

MODERATE DRINKING

A study done in 1926 found that moderate drinkers lived for two to five years longer than nondrinkers. Since then, dozens of studies have supported this claim. But scientific groups and governments differ on what moderate drinking means. After the American Cancer Society did a study of its own, it recommended a daily maximim of 10 ounces of wine (at 12 percent alcohol), 24 ounces of beer (at 5 percent), or 3 ounces of liquor (at 40 percent). Most authorities agree with this recommendation.

Examples of an average drink

A shot of spirits
1½ oz

A glass of wine
4 oz

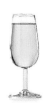

An aperitif
2 oz

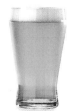

A pint of beer
16 oz

Other beneficial effects of red wine

Recent research has shown that the body may need naturally occurring chemicals called antioxidants to stay healthy. Red wine contains polyphenols, potent sources of antioxidants. The value of antioxidants is that they neutralize free radicals. These are molecules that oxidize harmful substances in the body but that can also run amok, turning on the body's own cells. A surfeit of these free radicals is thought to contribute to many degenerative diseases—including heart disease and cancer—and even hasten the aging process itself.

An unresolved debate

It has to be said, however, that the case for red wine is not entirely won. Although surveys point statistically to health benefits from drinking red wine, there is still the possibility that the benefits may have more to do with the character of red wine drinkers than with the wine itself. An ongoing study by Dr. Arthur Klatsky and his colleagues at the Kaiser Permanente Medical Center, Oakland, California, has found that wine drinkers are more likely than beer drinkers to be moderate in their consumption, to smoke less or not at all, and to be better educated about dietary matters.

Also, the Mediterranean way of drinking wine—in moderate quantities with meals consisting of the healthier diet of fresh vegetables, lean cuts of meat, and olive oil—may go further toward solving what many nutritional scientists have called the French Paradox. And it may actually be the foods wine drinkers eat that offer protection against heart disease (see page 114).

Although the potential benefits of red wine may seem appealing, they are not a rationale for excessive drinking. Rates of liver cirrhosis and other alcohol-related diseases are actually much higher in France

THE PERILS OF EXCESSIVE DRINKING

As reports of the benefits of moderate drinking increase, many people may ignore the dangers of excessive alcohol consumption. Alcohol slows reaction time and disrupts orientation, so operating machinery, driving, or crossing a road can be dangerous. But many people drink regularly without suffering too greatly from drunkenness and assume that their drinking is not harmful. If you regularly drink substantial amounts of alcohol, however, you may permanently damage your liver, heart, and brain, and may be increasing your risk of falling prey to certain cancers. Such fatal conditions as cirrhosis of the liver are directly related to alcohol consumption. In addition to its devastating long-term damage, alcohol immediately attacks several of the body's systems; this action is what causes the unpleasant effects known as a hangover.

THE BEST REMEDY
The first step after diagnosis of any alcohol-related health problem should be to stop drinking.

Depression
Heavy alcohol consumption gradually destroys the brain cells and can result in depression, memory loss, and intellectual deterioration.

Liver disease
Persistent and excessive consumption may lead to fatty liver, alcoholic hepatitis, cirrhosis, and liver cancer.

Digestive disorders
Heavy drinkers may suffer from digestive tract diseases such as gastritis, pancreatitis, and cancer of the upper digestive tract.

Nerve damage
Malnutrition, common among alcoholics, disturbs nerve functioning, causing symptoms such as cramps and numbness.

Mouth and throat cancer
High levels of alcohol intake increase the risk of cancers of the mouth, tongue, and throat.

Heart disease
Heavy drinkers are more susceptible to coronary heart disease and hypertension (high blood pressure) and are more likely to suffer a stroke.

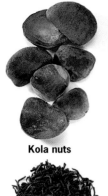

Kola nuts

Tea

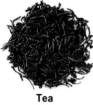

Cocoa beans

Coffee beans

CAFFEINE SOURCES
Plant products, such as tea, cocoa beans, kola nuts, and coffee beans, that contain caffeine are found all over the world.

than in the United States. And studies have shown that habitual teetotalers, such as Seventh Day Adventists, live healthy lives.

WOMEN AND ALCOHOL

How much alcohol in the body may be considered safe depends on such things as weight, age, diet, genetics, and illnesses suffered, but women in general should drink less alcohol than men. The reason is not just that women tend to have smaller frames proportionally but also that their bodies contain more fat, in which alcohol will not dissolve. And since women have less water in their bodies than men, their alcohol intakes do not become as diluted. Therefore, after a woman drinks the same amount of alcohol as a man, a higher concentration appears in her blood than in that of a man of the same weight. This makes women more prone to liver disease. Some research also suggests that excessive alcohol consumption increases the risk of breast cancer.

Drinking during pregnancy

Alcohol can cause fetal alcohol syndrome (FAS). FAS was first identified in the mid-1970's by researchers at the University of Washington who studied birth defects and growth abnormalities among babies of women who drank heavily. FAS can lead to the baby being born with such maladies as a harelip, cleft palate, flattened face, heart defects, deformed limbs, and mental retardation. Such babies also tend to suffer growth retardation and poor muscle function.

Some researchers claim that as little as one drink a day during pregnancy can cause low birthweight in babies; the equivalent of two glasses of wine per day can produce a 1 in 10 chance of FAS.

Doctors advise women not to drink at all while they are trying to conceive or during the crucial first 12 weeks of pregnancy. However, many doctors acknowledge that a few glasses of wine taken before confirmation of pregnancy is unlikely to do harm.

THE HIGHS AND LOWS OF CAFFEINE

Caffeine has become an indispensable part of modern living. Almost everyone gets a lift from a morning cup of tea or coffee, and all age groups are avid consumers of caffeine, since in addition to coffee and tea, it is present in colas and other soft drinks, cocoa, and chocolate.

The ability of caffeine to increase alertness and ward off sleep is well known. Long-distance truck drivers, night workers, and students studying for exams welcome the lift a cup of coffee or tea brings. Not only does it prevent sleepiness, it actually helps the thought processes become clearer, sharpens sensory perception, and improves reaction time. After only two cups of coffee (or the equivalent), driving skills may improve. Caffeine also prevents lapses of concentration and reduces irritability. It is popular with dieters because it raises the basal metabolic rate (the rate at which heat is produced when the body is at rest), so that calories are burned more quickly.

CAFFEINE LEVELS IN DIFFERENT DRINKS

A 5-fluid-ounce cup of brewed coffee contains about 80 milligrams of caffeine. This figure means little, however, unless it is compared with the caffeine levels in other drinks. An equal cup of instant coffee, for example, contains approximately 65 milligrams, and decaffeinated coffee, only 3 milligrams per cup. On average, brewed tea contains about 60 milligrams of caffeine. Cocoa and chocolate drinks have about 5 milligrams of caffeine per cup.

A CUP OF CAFFEINE
The level of caffeine in a cup of coffee, tea, or cocoa can vary enormously. The amount of caffeine in tea also depends on how long it is brewed. Cola drinks usually vary from 30 to 60 milligrams per 12-ounce can, but decaffeinated colas are available.

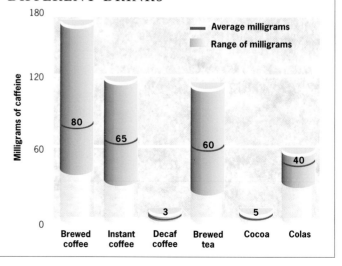

Adverse effects

The bad news is that drinking cup after cup of coffee or tea may be harmful to your health. Large doses of caffeine can make the heart beat faster and cause irregular beats. For this reason caffeine has been linked to an increased risk of high blood pressure.

For dieters caffeine is a mixed blessing, since in addition to burning off calories, it also stimulates the release of insulin, which causes blood sugar to drop, creating feelings of hunger. So caffeine is only an aid to weight loss if the dieter can successfully ignore the hunger pangs that follow.

Too much coffee may result in tremors and sleeplessness. People who habitually drink up to 12 cups of strong coffee a day complain of symptoms ranging from sweating to anxiety. These symptoms disappear after just 36 hours without drinking coffee. People who suffer gastric irritation or ulcers should avoid caffeine because it stimulates acid secretion in the stomach.

Children and caffeine

Growing children are also at risk from caffeine. Although they tend not to drink much tea or coffee, they do consume cola drinks that contain the drug. Because children are smaller than adults, they take in proportionally more caffeine from each cola and it therefore has a greater effect. One can of cola for a child may be the equivalent of four cups of coffee for an adult. Many countries now limit the caffeine level in colas and other soft drinks, but caffeine-free beverages may be better for children.

DECAFFEINATING COFFEE

Concern about the safety of chemicals used for decaffeinating coffee has led to the development of various water methods. For example, the Swiss water method retains most of the bean's taste by soaking beans in flavor-charged water. A more common water method is shown below.

Extracting coffee
Water is run through the green beans to produce a coffee extract.

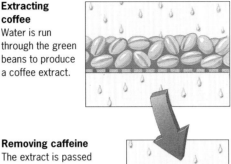

Removing caffeine
The extract is passed over an activated carbon (charcoal) filter that absorbs the caffeine.

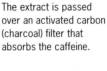

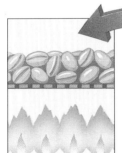

Adding flavor
The flavor, which was removed during the process, is added, and the product is dried.

HINTS ON CUTTING DOWN

It's best to limit your daily intake of caffeine to 200 to 250 milligrams or about three cups of brewed coffee. Gradually reducing your caffeine intake, rather than suddenly stopping, will help to prevent withdrawal symptoms such as headaches, lethargy, and irritability.

▶ *If you normally drink coffee or tea from a mug, switch to a smaller cup.*

▶ *Change from ground coffee to instant.*

▶ *Drink decaffeinated coffee every other cup.*

▶ *Mix decaffeinated coffee with regular to reduce total caffeine intake.*

▶ *Swap your strong tea for a weak one.*

▶ *Brew the tea for a shorter time than usual.*

▶ *Drink decaffeinated colas and other sodas.*

COFFEE SUBSTITUTES

When cutting down your caffeine intake, be aware that you may be replacing your caffeine-rich drinks with something worse. Many soft drinks have high sugar levels, colorings, and preservatives. But there are also dangers in drinking some herbal teas, once thought to be the ideal substitute for coffee. A popular tea made from the roots of the kava plant is associated with hallucinations and dimmed vision. Another tea is made from the root bark of the sassafras tree, which has been linked with depression and hypothermia. Of course, many herbal teas are harmless; check with an herbalist to be sure.

HEALTHY BREW
Some herbal teas, such as rosehip, chamomile, mint, and vervain, are usually safe to drink in moderation. Alternatively, drink hot water flavored with fresh lemon or lime. Fruit drinks that are brewed in hot water are also an enjoyable substitute for coffee.

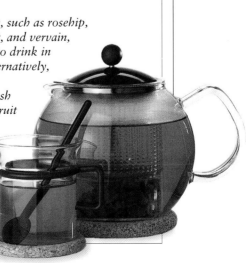

Juicy goodness

Blend your own fruits and vegetables for delicious liquid refreshments and concentrated goodness.

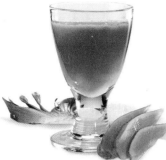

SOOTHING INDIGESTION
Papaya and pineapple juices may help to ease indigestion. Their enzymes—papain in papaya and bromelain in pineapple—ease pain in the upper abdomen.

PREVENTING CANCER
A red pepper and carrot cocktail is rich in sources of the antioxidants beta carotene and vitamin C.

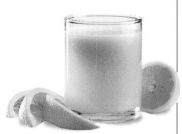

ABSORBING IRON
Fresh citrus juices make ideal accompaniments to meals. They contain plenty of vitamin C, which helps the body to absorb iron from foods.

THE JOYS OF JUICE

Drinking of fruit and vegetable juices has become much more prevalent in recent years. Many people start each day with a glass of freshly squeezed orange juice, while others harvest their own crops of fruits and vegetables to press themselves, or follow diet regimens that are based on juices.

The health benefits

Most fruits and vegetables are excellent sources of the antioxidants vitamins A and C, plus phytochemicals. These nutrients and chemicals, research suggests, help to neutralize harmful effects of the body's free radicals, which have been linked to aging, heart disease, and cancer (see page 94).

Juices can also make you feel healthier because they contain plant enzymes that aid digestion. It is even claimed that juices are able to alleviate many common complaints such as sore throat and insomnia. But fruit juices such as apple and citrus juices naturally contain about 10 percent sugar and, if consumed frequently throughout the day, will cause tooth decay.

Making your own

Although juices do not pack as much of a punch nutritionally as raw, fibrous fruits and vegetables do, they are often tastier. Carrot juice is a notable example. Juices are also a good way to boost your vitamin intake. In most cases a glass of fresh juice provides several times the recommended levels of vitamins and minerals, and because they are water based, the body will excrete any excess.

Freshly squeezed juices are better than store-bought juices because vitamin C diminishes with time and with exposure to air. They are also more likely to be free of any additives. Citrus fruits can be squeezed by hand, but with a juicing machine you can make a variety of cocktails. Thoroughly wash all vegetables and fruits you use to remove traces of insecticides and fertilizers.

Ready-made juices

Many manufacturers add preservatives and additives to packaged or bottled juice. Often, however, these are naturally occurring plant by-products and not necessarily harmful. By far the most common ingredient added to juice is refined sugar.

If you buy ready-made juices or frozen concentrates, read the labels to make sure that they have no added sugar or colorings, especially if you are giving them to children. For younger children, even pure fruit juices should always be diluted; many juices are acidic and can damage young teeth or cause diarrhea if children drink them at full strength.

JUICES AND THEIR NUTRIENTS

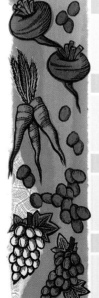

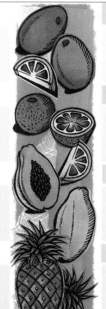

BEET (COOKED)
Folic acid, magnesium, potassium, calcium, iron.

CARROT
Beta carotene, folic acid, potassium, magnesium, phosphorus.

CRANBERRY
Vitamin C, potassium.

GRAPE
Vitamin C (if fortified), magnesium, potassium.

MANGO
Beta carotene, vitamin C, magnesium, potassium.

ORANGE
Vitamin C, beta carotene, folic acid, magnesium, phosphorus.

PAPAYA
Vitamin C, beta carotene, phosphorus, potassium.

PINEAPPLE
Vitamin C, folic acid, magnesium.

CHAPTER 7

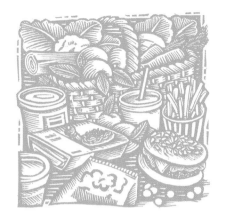

HEALTHY AND HARMFUL FOODS

*In the past few years, there has been
a growing awareness, backed by worldwide
research, that certain kinds of food may
protect against disease or form part of a cure,
whereas an excess of other foods can contribute to problems such as cancer, heart disease,
obesity, and tooth decay. At the same time,
new farming, processing, and packaging
techniques plus increased consumption of
convenience foods and fast foods have
raised new concerns about the health
consequences of the food we eat.*

THE FRESHNESS FACTOR

In today's marketplace many foods have been processed or packaged to give them a longer shelf life or make them more convenient to use. How safe or valuable are these processes?

THE FRESHEST WAY

Although the nutritional value of fresh produce diminishes between harvesting and sale, you can still get the best from your food if you

▶ *Shop for fresh produce frequently rather than once a week.*

▶ *Buy local produce that is in season.*

▶ *Use vegetables and fruits as soon as possible. If you cannot use them immediately, store root vegetables and onions, unwashed, in a dark, well-ventilated cupboard. Store other vegetables in the refrigerator.*

SCRUBBING VEGETABLES The peel and the layer under it contain valuable nutrients, so scrub vegetables clean rather than peeling them. But do cut green spots from potato peels.

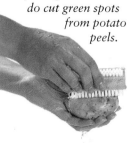

Foods are treated in various ways to prevent decay. They may be subjected to heat or cold, drying, irradiation, or chemical processes to slow spoilage and make them available at great distances from their growing source or despite seasonal fluctuations. Although surveys show that many people are making an effort to use fewer processed foods and more fresh ones, it has been estimated that ready-to-eat foods still make up between 75 and 80 percent of most people's diets in the United States.

The concern over processed foods is that they may not provide a well-balanced diet because of what is lost or added during processing. Many manufacturers and fast-food chains are aware of these concerns today and are striving to make their wares more healthful by cutting salt or fat or offering greater selections of fruits and vegetables and whole-grain products.

MISSING NUTRIENTS

During processing, foods lose some of their vitamins and minerals. For example, when vegetables and fruits are heated as part of the canning process, their B and C vitamins are reduced. Although minerals are not affected by heating, they are often leached into the canning liquid. Up to 50 percent of minerals such as magnesium and zinc can be lost if the canned liquid is not consumed or added to soups or stews. Canned vegetables lose even more vitamins if they are stored

NUTRITIONAL CONTENT OF FRESH AND PROCESSED FOODS

PRODUCT	QUANTITY	CALORIES	PROTEIN (grams)	CARBOHYDRATE (grams)	FAT (grams)	SODIUM (milligrams)
CHICKEN						
Roasted with skin	4 oz	270	28	0	17.5	90
Roasted without skin	4 oz	185	31	0	7	101
Canned	4 oz	260	14	0	20	1,216
PEACH						
Fresh	1 medium	37	0.6	9.7	0.1	3
Canned slices	2 oz	52	0	14	0	2
Frozen slices	2 oz	118	0.8	30	0.2	8
POTATO						
Boiled	4 oz	82	2	20	0.1	8
Canned	4 oz	72	1.7	17	0.1	287
Dried flakes, rehydrated	4 oz	81	2.3	18	0.1	299
PEAS						
Fresh	4 oz	95	8	8	1.7	trace
Canned	4 oz	92	6	15.5	1	288
Frozen	4 oz	80	6.9	11	1	2.5

for more than a year, unless the storage temperature is cooler than 65°F. The canning process, however, effectively protects us from microbes that cause food poisoning.

Another way in which nutrients are lost is through milling, or refining, of grain. During this process the bran and germ, which contain most of the B vitamins and minerals, are removed. Although today many refined breads and breakfast cereals are fortified with some of the nutrients that have been taken away during milling, the end product never quite matches the original grain nutritionally, and the fiber is irretrievably lost.

Sometimes the problem with processed food is not only what has been lost but what has been added. Many manufactured products tend to have unhealthful levels of salt, sugar, or fat, especially saturated fat. The only way to determine just what these levels are is to read labels carefully. Manufacturers are required to list the ingredients in the order of their quantity by weight.

HOW FRESH IS "FRESH" FOOD?

There is a difference between garden-fresh and market-fresh foods. Produce that is sold as "fresh" may not be as wholesome as it appears. Much "fresh" fruit comes from abroad or from across the country and has spent days or weeks in transit and storage. Even locally harvested vegetables are often stored before being sold. The moment a fruit or vegetable is picked, it starts losing nutrients because it continues to respire and exhaust its nutrient supply. Ideally, fruits and vegetables should be eaten the same day they are harvested. Unfortunately, this is rarely possible unless you grow your own.

Frozen fruits and vegetables, however, can be just as nutritious as fresh. Because they are usually harvested at peak quality and quick-frozen, they retain nearly all of their food value. In fact, fruit that is frozen shortly after picking may keep more of its vitamin C than fresh fruit that is in transit or storage for long periods.

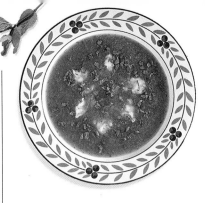

QUICK AND NOURISHING
A tasty pea soup for two can be made with 4 oz of frozen peas, 1 chopped small onion, ½ small head of lettuce, chopped, 1 tbsp chopped mint, 1 tsp olive oil, 1/4 tsp salt, 2 cups water, and a topping of 1 tbsp plain yogurt. This compares favorably with canned pea soup except that 8 oz of this fresh soup has only 403 mg of sodium, while 8 oz of canned soup has 895 mg.

PROCESSED FISH

An important source of protein and other nutrients in the diet, fish is not always available fresh. Many species are caught far from where they are consumed, and these are processed for preservation in a variety of ways. Most canned fish are preserved in vegetable oils that are low in saturated fats (see page 52).

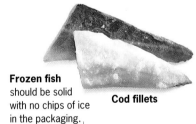

Frozen fish should be solid with no chips of ice in the packaging.

Cod fillets

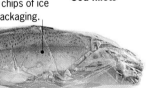

Trout

Choose canned fish that are packed in water if you are concerned about the fat content of your diet.

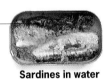

Sardines in water

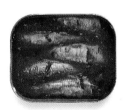

Sardines in oil

Sardines in tomato sauce

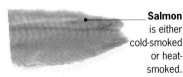

Haddock

Fish stays uncooked when it is cold-smoked.

Salmon is either cold-smoked or heat-smoked.

Salmon

FROZEN FISH
Frozen fish are not only quick and easy to cook but also retain much of their original nutritional value. Such fish are usually prepared and frozen on the fishing trawlers when they are in peak condition. Products include whole fish, fillets, breaded fish, shellfish, and ready-prepared dishes that need only reheating. When choosing frozen fish, look for discoloration—an indication that the fish may have thawed and been refrozen.

CANNED FISH
Some oil-rich fish and shellfish are preserved by canning—packed in oil, water, or tomato sauce. With their high protein content, canned sardines, salmon, tuna, crabmeat, and mussels provide nutritious meals or snacks. Oil-rich fish are a valuable source of omega-3 fatty acids, which help to reduce the risk of heart disease (see page 53). Eating canned salmon and sardines with their bones will provide a good intake of calcium.

SMOKED FISH
Certain fish, like haddock and salmon, are preserved by smoking; that is they are salted before being hung in an oven or kiln, where smoke from burning hardwood is blown over them for varying periods of time. The chemical properties of smoke are such that smoked fish should be consumed only occasionally. The salt content of smoked fish can vary (see label for amount) and may not be suitable for people on low-salt diets.

Dried fruit

For a ready supply of wholesome snacks, you can dry your own fresh fruit in an oven. Choose firm fruit that is just ripe. Leave berries whole, but peel, core, and thinly slice other fruits. To prevent fruits such as apples from darkening, coat them with a solution of ascorbic acid and water. A convection oven is preferred for drying because its fan will circulate the air. If you are using a conventional oven, prop open the door and set a fan nearby to blow air into the oven. Make sure the room is well ventilated. Keep the oven temperature between 120°F and 140°F. Place the fruit on baking sheets and rotate them from time to time. When the fruit is ready, it will feel malleable and leathery. Special dehydrators for fruit are also available.

GETTING IT RIGHT

If a diet high in processed foods is supplemented with several daily servings of fresh fruits and vegetables, the body probably gets all the nutrients it needs. But this does not mean that the diet is healthy or balanced —it may still contain too much fat, salt, and sugar and too little fiber, if whole-grain cereals and breads are omitted and too many high-fat snacks or desserts are consumed. But when time for shopping, preparing, and cooking fresh foods is limited, as it is for many people, processed foods may play a helpful role without posing a risk to good health. With careful selection, such processed foods as whole-grain crackers, canned sardines, and frozen vegetables, may be nutritionally sound as well as convenient.

PROCESSING AND PACKAGING

Food preservation methods include adding chemicals, drying, freezing, heating, irradiating, refining, and fermenting. Then the food is packed in anything from a steel or an aluminum can to a cardboard box or a plastic-wrapped container. There is some concern, however, that these processes damage the food they are designed to protect.

Irradiation

Of all the preserving techniques, irradiation has aroused the most fear. People are worried that the food may be radioactive and that it can be life-threatening. But, in fact, irradiated food is not radioactive, and the doses of radiation used to preserve them have been approved by the United Nations Joint Committee on Food Irradiation. Also, by law, all foods that have been irradiated must be labeled to indicate such.

Irradiation works by exposing food to a dose of gamma rays from a radioactive source. The rays kill up to 90 percent of disease-causing and other bacteria that occur naturally in many foods, preventing them from accumulating and producing toxins. Low doses of radiation can prevent sprouting in potatoes and onions. The technique also slows the ripening process in fruits and vegetables, thus increasin their shelf life.

Not all foods benefit from irradiation. Fats, for example, become more susceptible to rancidity. For this reason, irradiation is not used for most milk products and fatty or oily foods, such as sardines. Another important concern with irradiation is nutrient loss. Among vitamins that can be damaged are A, E, and K. Depending on the food, however, vitamin losses caused by irradiation are about the same as the losses from preparation and cooking.

Freezing

Freezing is one of the best ways to preserve the nutritional content of food. With vegetables and fruits, fewer nutrients are lost by freezing than with any other preserving

THE IRRADIATION OF FOOD

Irradiation of tomatoes and other fresh fruits and vegetables destroys bacteria, molds, and insects and delays ripening. It also prevents sprouting of potatoes, garlic, and onions and thus helps to maintain their freshness during distribution and storage.

INCREASING THE SHELF LIFE
To irradiate food, gamma rays from a radioactive source are directed onto packaged food. The rays pass through the food, splitting the DNA (genetic material) of the food's natural bacteria, thus killing the bacteria. Irradiation reduces the risk of food poisoning and extends the shelf life of fruit and vegetables by slowing the ripening process.

Fresh produce passes along a conveyor belt to irradiation chamber.

Gamma rays from a radioactive source are directed onto produce.

DNA is split by gamma rays.

DNA

Bacteria

Food particles

Bacteria are killed when DNA is split.

Irradiated food

method, especially when they are picked at the peak of ripeness and frozen immediately. Freezing stops the activity of bacteria and enzymes, which cause vitamin loss and decay, because the water in the food is bound as ice. However, the bacteria are not killed and can become active again when the food thaws; it should be used immediately.

Freezing can affect the texture of foods that are not rapidly frozen or are subjected to thawing and refreezing. Vegetables and fruits with a high water conent, should not be frozen at all, unless they have been cooked and finely chopped or pureed. Included in this group are potatoes, tomatoes, zucchini, cucumbers, and eggplant. Also cream and milk will separate when frozen.

Safe packaging

Some forms of packaging may taint food. In particular, fears have been raised over the safety of plastic wrap. Supermarkets and delicatessens sell many foods, such as meat, cheese, sandwiches, and fruits and vegetables wrapped in this stretchy polyvinyl chloride (PVC) product. Plasticizers are added to the PVC to make it cling, and the possibility of these plasticizers migrating into the wrapped foods causes concern.

The National Toxicology Program in the United States was the first to publish findings showing that plasticizers could cause cancer in test animals. Britain's Ministry of Agriculture, Fisheries and Food initiated research that revealed the plasticizer known as di-2-ethylhexyl, or DEHA—which is thought to cause cancer—was eight times more likely to end up in food than other plasticizers. Migration was at its worst in tightly wrapped high-fat products like salami, pork, and beef. The biggest absorption of plasticizers occurred with foods that had been wrapped in plastic wrap and then cooked in a microwave oven.

Although the threat to health posed by plastic wrap is not yet clear, avoid placing products containing DEHA in microwaves. If possible, purchase products that are labeled "Non-PVC" or "Plasticizer-free" or remove the food from store containers and rewrap in plastic bags at home.

Aluminum

Another suspect packaging material is aluminum. Research conducted in the United Kingdom and United States has shown that aluminum may be a danger to the elderly, particularly people with kidney disorders. It also may be a contributory factor in anemia and Alzheimer's disease. It is possible, but highly unlikely, that aluminum can enter the body through foods that are packaged in aluminum cans or cooked in aluminum foil or saucepans (see page 74).

ORGANIC PRODUCE

Fears about adulterated produce and the effects of intensive farming on the environment have led to the increasing popularity of organic, or "green," foods.

(see page 74).

USING PLASTIC WRAP SAFELY

Covering dishes of food to be cooked in a microwave oven will help to retain moisture. Steam will be produced that helps to speed the food's cooking time. Always use microwave-safe, non-PVC plastic wrap.

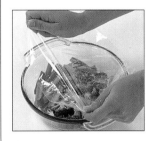

ALLOWING SPACE
When covering a dish with plastic wrap, do not let it touch the food.

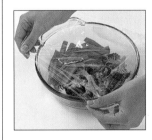

VENTING PLASTIC WRAP
Steam can split the plastic wrap, so turn back a corner to form an opening, which will allow steam to escape.

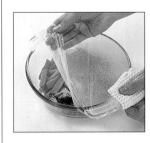

AVOIDING BURNS
To avoid getting burned when removing the plastic wrap, lift the edge farthest from you and then carefully peel it toward you.

DRYING METHODS

Originally, foods such as dates and grapes and strips of meat or fish were spread out in the sun to dry. Meat and fish were also smoked to dry them. Modern drying methods, however, are more varied and allow additional types of food to be preserved this way. Some vegetables and fruits are tunnel-dried—they are placed in a tunnel and exposed to hot blasts of air until their moisture content is reduced to 25 percent. Potatoes, milk, and eggs may be dehydrated until they retain only 2 to 10 percent moisture.

Accelerated freeze-drying involves a process that removes moisture from food after it has been frozen. This method is used to make instant coffee and freeze-dried fruits and vegetables used by campers and the military. The flavor and color of these products, when reconstituted, are often of good quality, comparing well to the fresh food.

DRIED FOODS
The oldest method of preserving food, drying removes water and thereby stops bacterial growth and inhibits enzyme activity.

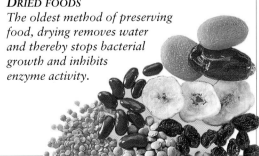

KEEPING ORGANIC FOOD SAFE

The possibility of lower chemical residues may make organic food safer to eat, but there are still some precautions needed when selecting, using, and storing such foods.

▶ *Look for a guarantee that the product has met stringent organic guidelines.*

▶ *Use fresh organic products as soon as possible after purchase. They spoil more quickly.*

▶ *Just before using them, wash all vegetables and fruits thoroughly under cold running water.*

▶ *Store food rich in nuts, seeds, and oils in the refrigerator rather than the cupboard to avoid rancidity. Do not keep them for more than a few weeks.*

▶ *Follow strict guidelines when canning or bottling produce, whether conventional or organic.*

Organic farmers raise crops without chemical fertilizers or pesticides. They instead use traditional techniques, such as mixed farming (planting two or more crops in the same field), crop rotation (planting different crops in sequence), shallow plowing, and fertilizing with animal manure, together with products like seaweed fertilizers and such methods as natural biological pest control. In any subsequent processing, no additives, preservatives, or irradiation are used.

Is organic food better?

Its supporters claim that organic produce is more nutritious, but numerous laboratory tests to compare the nutrients in organically and conventionally grown produce have not found substantial nutritional differences. They also profess that it is better for you because it contains no residues from pesticides and fertilizers. The jury is still out on this. Tests are being conducted on many of the chemicals used in intensive farming, and it is difficult to make definitive statements yet about the levels that are safe and the long-term effects on human health.

The regulation of pesticides

History, however, suggests there is some justification for concern about a few modern agricultural practices. The pesticide DDT was developed in the late 1930's and introduced in 1945. By 1972 it was outlawed in the United States after it was found to have damaging effects on the human nervous system. DDT was withdrawn from sale in Great Britain in 1984. Subsequently, all chemicals used in food production have come under scrutiny. However, DDT is still used in many developing countries that export fruits and vegetables.

Pesticide limits are strict in the United States. But in 1988 the National Academy of Science noted that "some allowed levels [of pesticide residues in food] are being challenged by scientists as being too high."

The U.S. Food and Drug Administration (FDA) routinely monitors the chemicals in foods. It maintains more than 10,000 regulations, including those for tolerance levels of 300 pesticides used by American farmers. Any farmer who exceeds the pesticide limits faces legal action, fines, and possibly the loss of his or her crops. But the FDA rarely discovers cases in which the pesticide tolerance levels are violated.

A few times a year, the FDA also does random tests on a variety of fresh and packaged foods from supermarkets all over the country. These foods are prepared and cooked as they would be for normal consumption. Then they are analyzed for pesticide residues with a standard that is five times below the legal tolerance limit. So far, the results from the FDA testings are positive. It seems that the majority of fruits and vegetables grown in the United States are well within tolerance limits and do not harbor unsafe levels of pesticides and other chemicals.

In spite of intense random checking of domestic and foreign produce, the FDA is unable to vouch for the safety of all foods

---

A DIFFERENT LOOK

Organic foods may please the palate, but they do not always tempt the eye because of blemishes and irregular shapes. They may also have insect residues (which should be washed off) and a strong aroma.

CONVENTIONAL PRODUCE
Many genetically altered foods are said to have a "designer look" that may appeal to consumers, but that does not ensure the food's nutritional value.

Apples are often waxed for a shiny appearance.

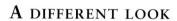

Pesticides used on conventional produce often leave residues on the outer surface.

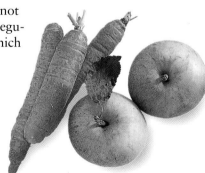

ORGANIC PRODUCE
The seeming imperfections of organic produce are harmless and do not affect the food's taste or nutritional value.

grown and sold in the United States, although the strict tolerance levels help to minimize the risk of eating contaminated food.

It is possible that the delayed effects on human health from synthetic pesticides and fertilizers are sufficiently small to be of no consequence. But until the investigations into all the modern farmer's chemical aids are complete, doubts may remain.

ARE THERE PERFECT FOODS?

To ensure a well-balanced diet, you normally need to eat a combination of foods. There are some foods, however, that contain such a wide range of essential nutrients that they may be considered almost perfect. Three such foods—wheat, bananas, and milk—are packed with so much goodness they seem to be in a class of their own.

WHEAT

Sometimes called the "staff of life," wheat provides anywhere from 15 to 60 percent of the calories and protein in most people's diets. Of the 44 known essential nutrients, only 5 are missing from wheat—vitamins A, B_{12}, C, and D, and iodine. The wheat berry contains 22 vitamins and minerals, protein, and dietary fiber but not in the quantities adequate for people. To get quality protein, wheat needs to be combined with a complementary protein food, such as dried beans and peas or nuts.

<table>
<tr><td>

CAUTION

Organic produce lacks the preservatives often present in those grown nonorganically, so always make sure the food is completely fresh. Moldy food (a major source of potent carcinogens) can pose a serious health risk.

</td></tr>
</table>

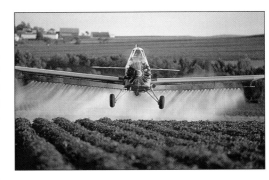

INTENSIVE FARMING
Fewer farmers now rely heavily on chemical fertilizers and pesticides. More of them are using integrated pest management with much lower applications of chemicals. Using chemical products, however, ensures a high crop yield and wards off spoilage, making food more widely available and cheaper for the consumer.

Is whole wheat better than refined?

The nutrients in wheat are not evenly distributed throughout the berry. Many of

ORGANIC WINE

A glass of wine can be even more enjoyable when it is low in artificial additives. It may be less likely to give you a reaction if you are sensitive to sulfites.

Organic wine is made from grapes grown without chemical fertilizers and pesticides. During wine making only low levels of sulfur dioxide are allowed, reducing the chances of an allergic reaction in people who suffer from asthma or bronchial problems.

To identify organic wines, look for an organic organization's symbol on the label. French bottles may also be labeled with a description such as *"Ce vin est cultivé sans engrais chimiques, sans insecticide"* or *"Production de l'agriculture biologique."*

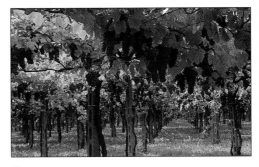

ORGANIC VINEYARD
Vines that are free from chemical fertilizers and pesticides can yield wines as high in quality as those from the most cultured grape. The quality of organic wines is as varied as that of ordinary wines. Their flavor and character are usually similar to conventionally produced wines from the same grape variety and region.

A grain of wheat

The wheat berry is a rich source of nutrients. The bran, five or six layers of protective coating, mainly consists of fiber. It also has a high proportion of B vitamins, some minerals, and protein. The germ of the wheat, which is the plant embryo, contains polyunsaturated fat, many B vitamins, vitamin E, and protein. The endosperm supplies food to the growing seed. It is mainly composed of starch granules and protein and has some B vitamins.

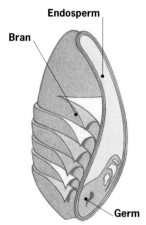

Endosperm

Bran

Germ

*UNREFINED WHEAT
The most nutritious whole-wheat flour is stone-ground, as it retains most of the original wheat berry.*

them are concentrated in the outer layers (bran) and in the germ (the tiny seed at the bottom of the kernel), both of which are lost when wheat is refined.

Refined wheat flour has 60 to 80 percent fewer nutrients than the whole kernel and only 10 percent of its fiber. Although manufacturers often fortify their cereals or breads with some of the vitamins and minerals that have been lost in the refining process and sometimes even a few not found in the original grain, the end product rarely matches the original nutritionally and never in fiber content. The fiber in wheat is important, because it helps to prevent constipation and perhaps reduce the risk of some cancers.

Is wheat fattening?

Wheat has suffered some bad publicity in the past. It was thought that its carbohydrate content made it fattening. The truth is that carbohydrates are an important energy source and are particularly valuable in the form of whole grains. Typically, a slice of bread has only 60 to 80 calories. It is not wheat itself but the creamy sauces, oily spreads, and butter that people put on bread and other wheat products, such as pasta, that add calories and contribute to obesity.

BANANAS

At 100 calories and almost no fat, a banana is an ideal between-meal snack and energy booster, as the many tennis players who eat them between sets can affirm. Bananas contain a large amount of potassium, a mineral that helps to control blood pressure and heart function, thus protecting against heart attack, stroke, and irregular heart rhythms. Bananas also contain 30 percent of the recommended daily requirement of vitamin B_6 and 20 percent of vitamin C.

MILK

Milk is an important source of nourishment at most ages of life. Essential for developing

children's bones and teeth, milk can also maintain health in adulthood and even into old age. It is a rich source of calcium and supplies other important minerals, notably zinc, magnesium, potassium, and phosphorus. Milk also contains high-quality protein and a wide range of vitamins—A, B_1, B_2, B_6, B_{12}, and, when fortified, D. Carbohydrate is present in the form of a disaccharide: lactose (milk sugar). Whole milk is also high in saturated fat, but by choosing low-fat or skim milk, you can enjoy the benefits of milk without going overboard on fat.

Although milk contains an abundance of many important nutrients, it is not a "complete" food. Milk lacks fiber and is a poor source of dietary iron and vitamin C. After the first few months of an infant's life, even breast milk needs to be augmented with other foods to produce a balanced diet.

The importance of calcium

Healthy growth and the maintenance of bones and teeth depend on a good supply of calcium (as well as zinc, copper, manganese, fluoride, and protein). Blood pressure is also influenced by calcium. American research has shown that children with the highest intake of calcium have the lowest blood pressure. Calcium is particularly important for girls and women. Adolescent girls who get little calcium may compromise the growth of their bone mass. In later life they are more apt to suffer from osteoporosis, a gradual thinning of the bone structure that may result in fractures. Pregnant and breast-

NUTRITIONAL CONTENT OF FLOUR (PER 4 OZ)

FLOUR	CALORIES	PROTEIN (grams)	CARBOHYDRATE (grams)	FAT (grams)	SODIUM (milligrams)	FIBER (grams)
Whole-grain	357	14.6	74	2.5	4	10.3
White (enriched)	395	10.8	89	1.5	4	4
Self-rising	380	10.2	87	1.5	414	4

WHAT MILK IS BEST?

Because of the differences in processing, milk differs in composition and nutritional value. Look at the label for help in choosing the right one for your diet. Most of the milk sold is pasteurized. Because the milk is heated to 162°F to kill bacteria, B vitamins are reduced by 10 percent and vitamin C by 25 percent.

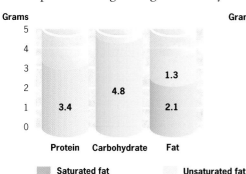

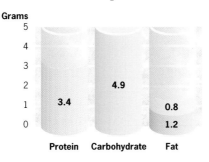

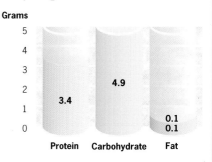

Saturated fat　　　　Unsaturated fat

WHOLE MILK
The average fat content of pasteurized whole milk is 3.3 percent. A 3.5-fluid-ounce portion of whole milk contains 3.4 grams of protein, 4.8 grams of carbohydrate, and 3.4 grams of fat, of which 2.1 grams are saturated.

LOW-FAT (2%) MILK
When milk is partly skimmed, it retains only a 2 percent fat content—it also loses a proportion of vitamin A and D content. A 3.5-fluid-ounce glass of low-fat milk contains 3.4 grams of protein, 4.9 grams of carbohydrate, and 2 grams of fat, of which 1.2 grams are saturated. Low-fat milk is not suitable for children under two years.

SKIM MILK
Milk that is skimmed has almost no fat—less than 0.5 percent. It retains the calcium of whole milk, but loses more vitamin A and D with the fat. A 3.5-fluid-ounce glass of skim milk contains 3.4 grams of protein, 4.9 grams of carbohydrate, and 0.2 gram of fat, of which 0.1 gram is saturated. Skim milk is not suitable for children under five years.

feeding women require calcium to support fetal and infant growth. During menopause, increased calcium intake may help to counteract the loss of bone mass resulting from reduced estrogen levels.

Children under the age of 11 should drink at least two to three cups of milk a day; teenagers and young adults, four cups; older adults, two to three cups; breast-feeding mothers and postmenopausal women, four cups or more. Choose low-fat milk for everybody over the age of five (see page 50).

Milk allergies
Not everyone can drink milk. Some people —especially Asians, Eskimos, Africans, Native Americans, and up to 40 percent of Caucasians—lack sufficient amounts of the enzyme lactase in their intestines to break down the lactose in milk (see page 108). For those people, milk with a reduced lactose content is available. Alternatively, lactose-intolerant persons can try eating yogurt, which has less lactose than milk but still contains plenty of protein and milk nutrients and is a more concentrated source of calcium (see page 102).

THE IDEAL FOOD
Breast milk is undoubtedly best for babies. It is free, does not need sterilizing, is the proper temperature, and contains just the right amount of proteins, vitamins, and minerals a growing baby needs.

In addition, breast milk contains important antibodies that provide the baby with a natural protection against viral illnesses, respiratory infection, and infections of the gastrointestinal tract.

Breast milk supplies the baby with 70 calories per 3.5 fluid oz.

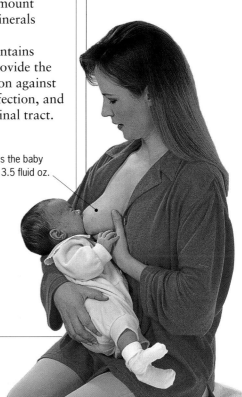

SATISFYING A BABY'S NEEDS
Breast milk provides a baby with essential nutrients. Some nutrients, such as iron and vitamin D, are absorbed much more efficiently from breast milk than from formula milk.

HEALTHFUL FOODS

Research has shown that some foods contain special nutrients, chemical compounds, and even bacteria that can help to prevent certain diseases, relieve health complaints, and boost energy.

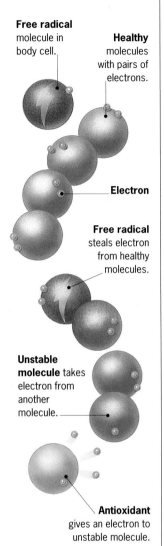

Free radical
molecule in body cell.

Healthy
molecules with pairs of electrons.

Electron

Free radical
steals electron from healthy molecules.

Unstable molecule takes electron from another molecule.

Antioxidant
gives an electron to unstable molecule.

FREE RADICALS AND ANTIOXIDANTS
Free radical molecules inside the body's cells sometimes attack other molecules by taking an electron. The healthy molecule in turn becomes a free radical and attacks another molecule, removing its electron. A chain reaction is started, which is broken when an antioxidant is present. The antioxidant, not requiring two electrons, offers one to the unstable molecule.

Evidence from more than 300 studies has revealed that fruits and vegetables offer powerful protection against disease. It appears that the vegetables with the most effective weapons against cancer and other diseases are the crucifers (so named because they have cross-shaped flowers), which include cabbage, broccoli, and cauliflower They contain antioxidants, which attack molecules called free radicals.

Free radicals are released in all cells as part of the body's normal biochemistry and defense mechanism against disease. They occur as a response to everyday living, for example, exposure to ultraviolet light waves and environmental pollutants such as motor vehicle emissions. If free radicals become too numerous, however, they attack the body itself. It is believed that unchecked free radical action can lead to premature aging and, through damage to DNA (genetic material), some forms of cancer.

THE BENEFITS OF ANTIOXIDANTS
Stable molecules in the body have pairs of electrons, while free radicals have at least one that is unpaired, making them unstable.

To achieve stability, free radicals steal electrons from other molecules, thereby making them unstable. The remaining molecule, which is now a free radical, sets off to take another electron from a complete molecule. A destructive chain reaction is thus set in motion. Antioxidants are substances that negate the harmful effects of free radicals by providing them with electrons, but do not themselves become unstable The antioxidants can then be safely broken down and absorbed by the body.

The main antioxidants are the carotenes, especially beta carotene (the plant source of vitamin A found in carrots and oranges); vitamins C and E; the minerals selenium, zinc, and magnesium; and protein, in particular glutathione, which is a combination of three amino acids—glutamate, glycine, and cysteine. These are found in the cruciferous family and many other fruits and vegetables, such as bananas and peas.

The antioxidants that have been subject to the most study are beta carotene, vitamin C, and vitamin E. In American trials, a high dietary intake of beta carotene has been associated with a reduced risk of both heart

---

HEALTHY HERB

Parsley is a member of the umbellifer family, which, like the crucifer family, is being investigated for its disease-fighting properties. This biennial plant contains beta carotene and vitamin C, which may protect against cancers and heart disease, and boost the immune system.

USING PARSLEY
There are several types of parsley, but the two best-known are curly-leafed parsley and flat-leafed (Italian) parsley. Parsley leaves offer B vitamins, iron, calcium, magnesium, and

fiber, as well as antioxidants. They can be added to a variety of dishes, including stews, salads, baked potatoes, and peas, or used as an edible garnish. Chewing raw parsley leaves can help to freshen breath.

Curly-leafed parsley

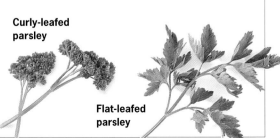

Flat-leafed parsley

disease and cancers of the mouth, throat, esophagus, larynx, lungs, stomach, cervix, and bladder. Other studies have uncovered a relationship between a high dietary intake of vitamin C, found in oranges and many other fruits and vegetables, and a reduced risk of cataracts, heart and brain disease, and nonhormonal cancers such as those of the stomach, lung, and throat. High consumption of vitamin E, found in vegetable oils and sunflower seeds, has been linked to a reduced risk of gastrointestinal cancer, lung cancer, and thrombosis (blood clots).

No match for nicotine

Antioxidants may help to protect the body from many illnesses, but they are no match for the effects of tobacco. A study of 29,000 long-term Finnish smokers, all over the age of 50, by the National Cancer Institute in the United States and Finland's National Public Health Institute found that regular doses of vitamin E and beta carotene did not lessen smokers' chances of suffering lung cancer or stroke. In fact, those who took the antioxidants had a higher incidence of these illnesses than a similar group of men who took nothing. The researchers were puzzled by these unexpected results and are still analyzing them. It is possible that cancer was already in progress and that antioxidants are preventive rather than therapeutic agents.

> ### CAUTION
> Some of the disease-fighting abilities of phytochemicals and antioxidants are destroyed by overcooking. To get the most good from vegetables, eat them raw, or lightly steamed, boiled, or microwaved.

PHYTOCHEMICALS

Discovered in 1978, phytochemicals are being hailed as the new hope in the ongoing fight against cancer. Phytochemicals—and there are literally thousands of them present in vegetables and fruits—are neither vitamins nor minerals but rather chemical compounds that evolved to protect plants from injury and disease. In humans, the phytochemicals seem to act as potent cancer inhibitors or as agents that can help to stimulate the body's natural mechanisms to inactivate noxious compounds. The cruciferous vegetables, noted for their antioxidant properties, are particularly rich in these chemicals, but other vegetables and fruits also contain important phytochemicals.

How do phytochemicals work?

Researchers in the United States found that if the phytochemical sulforaphane is added to human cells growing in a laboratory dish,

Anticancer foods

Phytochemicals and antioxidants are found in all fruits and vegetables. In addition to crucifers (the cabbage family), the following foods contain anticancer agents: corn, asparagus, carrots, peas, onions, garlic, celery, dates, figs, grapes, grapefruit, kiwifruit, bananas, oranges, pumpkins, soybeans, sweet potatoes, and tomatoes. Remember, a healthy diet should include at least five servings of fruits and vegetables every day.

PHYTOCHEMICALS

Sulforaphane, a phytochemical found in cruciferous vegetables, helps to prevent cells from developing cancer. It seems that within only hours of being eaten, sulforaphane enters the bloodstream and triggers a self-defense system in the body. This acts to detoxify carcinogens. Research is currently being carried out on developing a synthetic version of sulforaphane, but brussels sprouts are a prime natural source.

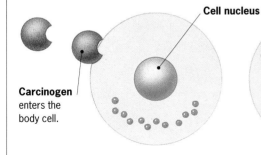

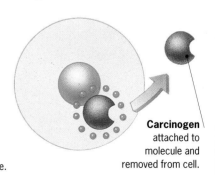

Cell nucleus

The phytochemical sulforaphane reaches the cell.

Carcinogen enters the body cell.

Phase 2 enzymes are activated by sulforaphane.

Carcinogen attached to molecule and removed from cell.

CARCINOGEN ATTACKS A CELL
The process of cancer development starts when a carcinogenic molecule or mutagen enters a cell.

DEFENSE MECHANISM IS TRIGGERED
When sulforaphane is introduced into the body, it activates phase 2 enzymes, which are naturally occurring cancer-fighting proteins in the cell.

THE CARCINOGEN IS REMOVED
The phase 2 enzymes attach the carcinogen to a molecule, which carries it away from the cell.

CANCER-PREVENTING VEGETABLES

Cruciferous vegetables and dark, leafy greens such as spinach are high in the antioxidants and phytochemicals that help fight cancer. Although cabbage and broccoli are perhaps the most well known of the crucifers, or cabbage family, other members include kohlrabi, turnip, rutabaga, mustard greens, kale, and collard greens. Most of these vegetables are available the year around but are at their best during the cold months.

	VEGETABLE	CHOOSING	STORING	USING
BROCCOLI				
	The star of the crucifer family, broccoli is rich in beta carotene, vitamin C, potassium, calcium, folic acid, and several phytochemicals.	The florets should be crisp and tightly closed. They should be a dark green or purplish color. Avoid any with brown or spotted stems.	Refrigerate, unwashed, in an open plastic bag. The broccoli will keep for about four days. Once cooked, store in a tightly covered container for up to three days.	Wash thoroughly under cold running water. Cut the stalks a few inches below the florets, and pierce the bottom of each stalk for even cooking.
BRUSSELS SPROUTS				
	Brussels sprouts are rich sources of sulforaphane and other phytochemicals and antioxidants. They are one of the best vegetable sources of dietary fiber.	The vegetables should be bright green and firm, with tight heads. Choose sprouts of a similar size for even cooking. Avoid any with yellow leaves.	Refrigerate, unwashed, in a perforated plastic bag for up to five days.	Rinse thoroughly. Trim stem ends. Cut an "X" in the bottom of each stem for even cooking.
CABBAGE				
	The many varieties of cabbage contain numerous antioxidant compounds. Chinese cabbage (bok choy) is a particularly rich source of beta carotene, vitamin C, potassium, and calcium.	Cabbage heads should have only three or four loose outer leaves that are pliable but not limp. Avoid heads with damaged leaves or split stems.	Refrigerate in a perforated plastic bag. An uncut cabbage will keep for about two weeks. Once cut, use within a couple of days.	Remove tough outer leaves. Cut the cabbage into quarters, then into wedges, before removing the core. For slicing, retain the core in the wedge to keep leaves from separating.
CAULIFLOWER				
	Cauliflower is rich in vitamin C, potassium, fiber, and several phytochemicals.	Cauliflower should have a firm white or creamy head. The outer leaves should be fresh green and crisp. Avoid heads with spots or loose florets.	Refrigerate, unwashed and stem side up, for up to five days. Ready-cut florets should be used within 24 hours of purchase.	Remove the leaves and cut out the core. Cook the head whole or separate into florets.
SPINACH				
	Spinach contains four times more beta carotene than broccoli and is a source of vitamins C and E. It is rich in fiber. But it contains oxalic acid, a chemical that limits the absorption of iron and calcium.	Leaves should be dark green, fresh, and crisp. Avoid spinach that is bruised or crushed. Stems should be thin.	Refrigerate, unwashed, in a plastic bag for up to four days.	Trim stems and wash thoroughly. Spinach that is to be cooked does not need to be dried; the water clinging to leaves will steam the spinach without additional cooking liquid.

it boosts the synthesis of cancer-fighting enzymes (protein substances that act as catalysts in the body, breaking down food and aiding metabolism). Like a policeman who removes a troublemaker from a peaceful gathering, these enzymes remove potential or actual mutagens and carcinogens from human cells by handcuffing them to a molecule and whisking them away before they can cause any lasting damage.

Phytochemicals use an impressive array of cancer-blocking tactics. Scientists at Cornell University in New York have reported that p-courmac and chlorogenic acid, two phytochemicals that are found in tomatoes as well as other fruits and vegetables, can prevent carcinogens from forming in the first place. Another anticancer tactic of phytochemicals is to close off the capillaries, hair-thin blood vessels, that deliver nutrients to developing tumors. But preventing existing cancers from spreading through the body is beyond the capability of these phytochemical compounds.

Fighting breast cancer

An overabundance of the hormone estrogen may stimulate the growth of breast cancer. But recent American research has shown that phytochemicals in food may help to beat this cancer by obstructing the body's absorption of estrogen. Widely prevalent in the United States, breast cancer may also be related to high intakes of fats that have combined with oxygen (oxidized).

A study by New York's Strang-Cornell Cancer Research Laboratory revealed that estrogen levels fell dramatically in women who consumed a diet high in cruciferous vegetables, such as cabbage, cauliflower, kale, and brussels sprouts. It is thought that one of the phytochemicals found in cruciferous vegetables—indole-3-carbinol—deactivates potent estrogens, thus preventing estrogen-sensitive cells, particularly those in the breast, from developing tumors.

Another potent phytochemical that has been linked to the prevention of breast cancer is sulforaphane (see box, page 95). Found in cruciferous vegetables, it also speeds up the removal of estrogen from the body.

Hope for the future?

Research into phytochemicals is still in its infancy, and there has not yet been time for long-term studies on humans to see whether an existing cancer can be retarded or eradicated by these compounds. According to scientists, phytochemical theory dovetails with the results of numerous studies that link diets rich in fruits and vegetables with a lower incidence of cancer. Besides fighting cancer, many phytochemicals show promise also in preventing heart disease and aging.

East and West

Women of all ages should include a range of cruciferous vegetables in their diets, eating plenty of cauliflower, cabbage, and brussels sprouts. Although postmenopausal women may no longer produce estrogen from their ovaries, there is still some present in body fat.

The traditional Japanese diet consists of large quantities of leafy green vegetables and is low in fat, and the incidence of breast cancer there has always been lower than in the West. More recently, however, the number of cases in Japan has risen dramatically—58 percent between 1975 and 1985. Some researchers believe that this rise is due to many Japanese people adopting a Western-style, high-fat diet.

CANCER AND DIET

Some scientists claim that a nutritionally deficient diet is a cause of many cancers. Three factors are thought to play a major role in increasing the possibility of developing cancer: low levels of antioxidants and fiber and high levels of certain kinds of fat.

CANCERS NOT ASSOCIATED WITH DIET
Scientists believe that the following cancers are caused by factors other than diet: brain (often from metastasis from breast or ovarian cancer), skin (too much sun and sunburn), and blood (leukemias).

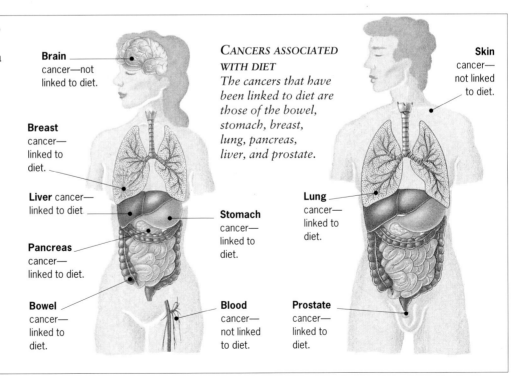

Brain cancer—not linked to diet.

Breast cancer—linked to diet.

Liver cancer—linked to diet

Pancreas cancer—linked to diet.

Bowel cancer—linked to diet.

CANCERS ASSOCIATED WITH DIET
The cancers that have been linked to diet are those of the bowel, stomach, breast, lung, pancreas, liver, and prostate.

Stomach cancer—linked to diet.

Blood cancer—not linked to diet.

Skin cancer—not linked to diet.

Lung cancer—linked to diet.

Prostate cancer—linked to diet.

Snacks for health

The best type of fruit or vegetable juice is undiluted, with no added sugar. All these drinks provide vitamins that act as antioxidants, and some berry drinks prevent bladder infections.

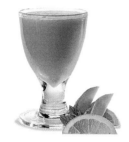

TROPICAL DELIGHT
Freshly squeezed orange juice, blended with mango, provides the antioxidants beta caroten and evitamin C and.

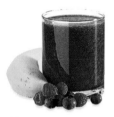

BERRY SURPRISE
Mix cranberries with a banana and some water and blend until smooth. Cranberry juice helps to prevent cystitis.

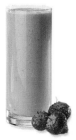

STRAWBERRY SHAKE
Strawberries combined with milk and plain low-fat yogurt provide a rich blend of vitamin C and calcium.

NEW WONDER FOODS

Cystitis, herpes, infertility—these three conditions affect thousands of men and women. Could the cure lie in simple foods that can be picked in a garden or gathered at the seashore? Over the past few years, there have been many studies to learn whether certain foods have healing properties. In particular, great claims have been made for cranberries, kelp, and strawberries.

WHAT CAN CRANBERRY JUICE DO?

Drinking a glass of cranberry juice regularly can help to prevent cystitis, a painful urinary infection that has a tendency to recur. The cause of cystitis is the *Escherichia coli* (*E. coli*) bacterium. Usually existing in the intestines, it can creep into the urinary tract where it sticks to the bladder cells and spreads infection. Symptoms include pain on urination and a frequent need to pass water, as well as abdominal pain and fever. More women than men suffer cystitis because the opening to the female urethra is closer to the anus, making it easier for bacteria to enter from the rectal area.

CYSTITIS

One of the main causes of cystitis is *E. coli* bacteria, which normally live harmlessly in the rectum, intestines, and on anal skin. It also may be caused by friction on the urethra.

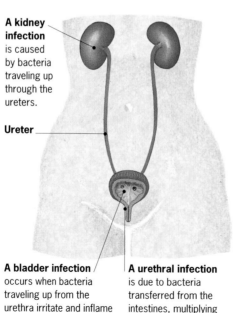

A kidney infection is caused by bacteria traveling up through the ureters.

Ureter

A bladder infection occurs when bacteria traveling up from the urethra irritate and inflame the lining of the bladder.

A urethral infection is due to bacteria transferred from the intestines, multiplying quickly in the urethra.

Cranberries have long been used by women as a folk remedy for cystitis. It was thought that the vitamin C in cranberries made the urine more acidic, thereby destroying the bacteria. Then in 1991, Israeli scientists at the Weizmann Institute of Science discovered two compounds in cranberry juice that cripple the mechanism by which the *E. coli* bacteria attach themselves to the walls of the urinary tract. Denied a firm hold, the bacteria are washed out in the urine, giving the infection no chance to flourish.

How much cranberry juice?

It appears that daily ingestion of 4 to 16 fluid ounces (½ cup to 2 cups) of cranberry juice can protect against the *E. coli* infection in people susceptible to cystitis. A study involving 72 postmenopausal women found that they were 58 percent less likely to develop bladder infections if they drank 10 fluid ounces of cranberry juice every day.

In another study, Prodromos N. Papas of the Tufts University School of Medicine in Boston found that drinking 16 fluid ounces (1 pint) of cranberry juice a day for three weeks helped to protect 73 percent of the group from recurring infections. When the women in the study stopped drinking the juice, half of them suffered a recurrence of the infection within six weeks. Drinking as little as 4 to 6 fluid ounces of cranberry juice a day may be enough to protect against cystitis, however. This amount prevented bladder infections in 19 out of 28 elderly women and men who took part in a 1991 study.

Although cranberry juice effectively prevents bladder infections or their recurrence, it should not be used for treating existing infections. If the symptoms are masked, the infection may spread to the kidneys and cause serious problems. If you develop cystitis, stop taking cranberry juice and seek medical advice for its treatment.

KELP AND HERPES

Those people unlucky enough to have contracted genital herpes are told that the condition is incurable and they will suffer recurring attacks throughout their lifetime. The severity of these attacks, however, could be minimized and possibly even prevented entirely if recent discoveries in test tube studies of kelp prove just as effective in human trials.

What can kelp do?

Researchers at the University of California put extracts of edible seaweed from the red algae family—generically known as kelp—into test tubes that contained human cells infected with the herpesvirus. The spread of the virus slowed by 50 percent. Also, human cells that were exposed to the kelp extract before being put in with the herpesvirus were immune to the infection.

It is not yet known what specific chemical component in kelp helps to destroy the herpesvirus. Kelp contains 13 vitamins, 20 amino acids, 24 trace elements, and many phytochemicals. Traditionally it has been used to treat a variety of complaints, particularly respiratory ailments, digestive disorders, and peptic ulcers. But there are health warnings about taking excessive amounts of kelp, as it can damage the thyroid gland.

Kelp is available as a supplement in both tablet and powder forms. The powder can be mixed with water for drinking or used as a salt substitute. It has a very strong flavor because of its iodine content.

STRAWBERRIES AND SPERM PRODUCTION

According to the latest research on vitamin C intake and healthy sperm, men who are trying to have children may reap benefits from eating strawberries and other fruits and vegetables that contain vitamin C. Just 200 milligrams a day—the amount found in 2½ cups of fresh strawberries—can restore sperm production and viability.

What causes unhealthy sperm?

Falling sperm counts among Western men have been worrying scientists in recent years. Modern-day pollutants and improper diet are among the main causes of low counts. Persistent exposure to toxic compounds, such as those found in air that has been polluted by petrochemicals, can result in those toxins accumulating in the testicles, where the sperm are produced. This can lead to sperm agglutination—a condition in which the sperm clump together after ejaculation and cannot move around freely—and contributes to infertility. Older men are particularly prone to this condition. A study comparing the sperm of 45-year-old men to that of 18-year-olds found that the older men had fewer, less mobile sperm with a higher incidence of malformation.

ORIENTAL MUSHROOMS

Cooks love mushrooms because they add delightful texture and flavor to many dishes. Health-conscious consumers appreciate them for other properties, especially the fact that they are fat free and low in calories (½ cup contains only 10 calories). They provide moderate amounts of calcium, potassium, and selenium, along with modest quantities of niacin and vitamin C.

Japanese studies have shown that mushrooms may favorably influence the immune system, with potential benefits in fighting cancer, infections, and such autoimmune diseases as lupus and rheumatoid arthritis. In addition, tree-ear mushrooms, used in many Chinese dishes, inhibit blood clotting. This quality may prove valuable in treating certain heart diseases.

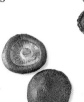

COOKING MUSHROOMS
Dried mushrooms add a wonderful rich, smoky flavor to cooked dishes. Soak them for about 30 minutes in a bowl of hot water before using them in soups or sauces.

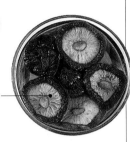

Reconstitute dried mushrooms before using them.

What can berries and vitamin C do?

A 60-day trial on infertile men carried out by Dr. William A. Harris at the University of Texas showed that a daily dose of 1,000 milligrams of vitamin C restored fertility to all of the men in the study. Their sperm counts rose by 60 percent; sperm were 30 percent livelier, and there were few abnormal sperm. Further tests by Dr. Harris and his colleagues showed that just 200 milligrams of vitamin C could produce the same results, although less quickly.

Scientists believe vitamin C is effective against sperm agglutination because of its powerful antioxidant effect. One theory suggests that free radical molecules in the body can attack the protective coating on the sperm's surface causing it to oxidize. The oxidized coating allows the sperm to clump together, which impedes their movement. Vitamin C increases the body's supply of antioxidants, which help to disable the free radicals (see page 94).

There is no conclusive proof, however, that vitamin C cures male infertility. Factors other than diet may pertain and men with this condition should not rely solely on an increased intake of vitamin C, whether from foods or supplements, to enhance function, but should seek medical advice.

STUPENDOUS STRAWBERRIES
As well as being a potent supplier of vitamin C, strawberries contain a natural substance called ellagic acid (also found in other berries, nuts, and a number of vegetables), which counteracts carcinogens and helps to prevent tumors from developing.

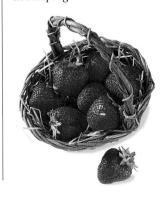

THE ENERGY BOOSTERS

Sugar to boost the body, caffeine to boost the mind—an all-too-familiar response to physical and mental tiredness. But do sugar and caffeine really help or are they actually counterproductive?

Glucose, a simple sugar derived from the carbohydrates in foods, is the body's preferred source of energy. Carbohydrates that are not immediately needed to fuel activity or metabolism are converted into glycogen, then stored in the liver and muscles. If insufficiently supplied with carbohydrates, the body can convert fat or protein to glucose.

Energy from sugar

Carbohydrate comes in two forms: simple, the sugars, and complex, the starches. Refined sugar (sucrose) is a simple carbohydrate. Whether it is brown or white table sugar, molasses, or in a syrup, sucrose provides a quick energy boost. But it provides energy with no nutritional support.

Natural sources of simple sugars (glucose, fructose, and maltose) include fruits and milk. These foods offer vital nutrients as well as an immediate supply of energy.

Unlike simple sugars, complex carbohydrates break down slowly in the body and supply glucose at a steadier rate. And like natural sources of simple sugars, complex-carbohydrate foods provide vitamins, minerals, and fiber (see page 46). Popular sources of complex carbohydrates include breads, pasta, rice, and potatoes.

Energy from caffeine

A cup of coffee or tea is widely used to offset the somnolent effects of a heavy meal. There is proof, at least with coffee drinking, that this antidote to the sleep-inducing effects of food actually works. Tests conducted by psychologists at the University of Wales College, Cardiff, on 32 men and women, found that coffee did indeed counteract after-meal lethargy by boosting alertness.

Considering that caffeine is a powerful stimulant both mentally and physically (see box below), this is hardly surprising. New research suggests that caffeine's energizing properties are due to its structural resemblance to a biochemical—adenosine—that calms some of the brain's activity when it is secreted there. If caffeine is present, your

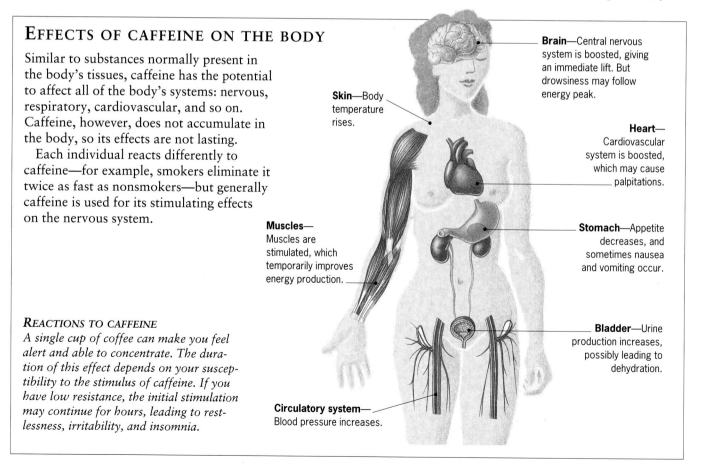

EFFECTS OF CAFFEINE ON THE BODY

Similar to substances normally present in the body's tissues, caffeine has the potential to affect all of the body's systems: nervous, respiratory, cardiovascular, and so on. Caffeine, however, does not accumulate in the body, so its effects are not lasting.

Each individual reacts differently to caffeine—for example, smokers eliminate it twice as fast as nonsmokers—but generally caffeine is used for its stimulating effects on the nervous system.

REACTIONS TO CAFFEINE
A single cup of coffee can make you feel alert and able to concentrate. The duration of this effect depends on your susceptibility to the stimulus of caffeine. If you have low resistance, the initial stimulation may continue for hours, leading to restlessness, irritability, and insomnia.

Skin—Body temperature rises.

Muscles—Muscles are stimulated, which temporarily improves energy production.

Circulatory system—Blood pressure increases.

Brain—Central nervous system is boosted, giving an immediate lift. But drowsiness may follow energy peak.

Heart—Cardiovascular system is boosted, which may cause palpitations.

Stomach—Appetite decreases, and sometimes nausea and vomiting occur.

Bladder—Urine production increases, possibly leading to dehydration.

brain's receptor sites will choose it rather than the adenosine and you will remain in a state of alertness.

Other researchers claim that caffeine is only effective as a booster in the short term, much like a stimulant drug. They say that the initial burst of energy quickly dissipates, leaving the muscles tired.

Natural energizers

Another brain energizer is a naturally occurring compound called choline. A component of acetylcholine, a neurotransmitter, choline in supplemental doses may help relieve some neurologic and psychiatric illnesses. Research undertaken on Alzheimer's disease by Dr. Richard J. Wurtman, a neuroscientist at the Massachusetts Institute of Technolgy, suggests that increased levels of choline can enhance memory and revitalize brain cells. Although choline is not a cure, adequate levels of it may help prevent the disease, and further research is under way.

A prime source of choline is lecithin—plentiful in egg yolks, sunflower seeds, and foods made from soy beans, such as tofu. Granulated lecithin, available in health food stores, can be used as a dietary supplement. However, most people do not need supplements, and excessive amounts of lecithin can cause gastrointestinal disturbances.

THE STONE AGE DIET

Since the modern diet of refined carbohydrates and plentiful fat is associated with many maladies, some people have gone back to the Stone Age—in dietary terms. The popular image of prehistoric humans is of successful hunters who feasted on freshly killed meat. But hunting was difficult, dangerous, and not always successful, so many of the foods our ancient ancestors depended on were nuts, fruits, roots, and vegetables gathered from the wild.

A study of 58 modern hunter-gatherer societies found that about two-thirds of them rely on plants rather than animals for their food. Research by A. S. Truswell, of the University of Sydney, on the !Kung tribe of South Africa revealed a generally healthy group of people whose diet was about 80 percent vegetarian. They did not exhibit the harmful effects associated with a Western diet, such as obesity, high blood pressure, and heart disease.

Adopting a simple diet

Advocates of the Stone Age diet recommend eating more nuts, seeds, and berries. They say that the distinctive ingredients of the contemporary diet—such as refined grain and dairy products, along with coffee, tea, alcohol, tobacco, and refined sugars—are the cause of most degenerative Western diseases, as well as many allergies. They are not, however, suggesting that nuts, seeds, and berries should be the only foods eaten. A balanced, healthy diet would be impossible with such a limited choice. The idea behind the Stone Age diet is to adopt it for a short time until the body cleanses itself, then to reintroduce other foods one by one while keeping watch for any allergic reactions.

Of course, not everyone wants to return to the Stone Age, even for a short visit, but that is no reason to miss out on the nutritional and health benefits that these "original" foods offer.

CHOOSING AND STORING NUTS

Nuts add variety, texture, and nutritional value to sweet and savory dishes. Here are some tips for getting the best from them.

▶ *To be sure of freshness, always buy from a shop with a high turnover.*

▶ *Whenever possible, buy nuts in their shells—shelled nuts become rancid quickly because of their high fat content.*

▶ *Reject shells with cracks, holes, or signs of mold.*

▶ *If a nut rattles in its shell, it is probably old (except for peanuts, which are legumes, rather than nuts).*

▶ *Store nuts in the freezer or in airtight jars in a cool, dry place.*

FOODS OF AN EARLIER AGE

Nuts and seeds are portable, tasty, and great energy sources because of their high fat content including omega-3 fatty acids. In addition to protein (10 to 25 percent by weight), they offer B vitamins; vitamin E; the minerals iron, calcium, potassium, and magnesium; and fiber—all of which are essential for good health.

Berries are also very nutritious. They are a good source of vitamin C, and some, like raspberries and blackberries, are high in fiber. Others have medicinal properties.

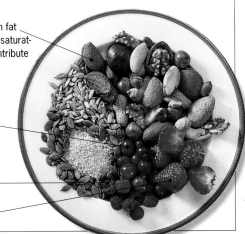

Nuts and seeds have a high fat content. The fat is mostly unsaturated and is not believed to contribute to atherosclerosis.

Cranberries have strong antibiotic and antiviral properties.

Raspberries contain salicylates, natural salts that have anti-inflammatory properties.

Strawberries contain natural antioxidants.

Yogurt

An ancient food, yogurt has had many great claims made about its healing properties, particularly its ability to fight certain kinds of infections. It is also a valuable source of important nutrients and, incidentally, is very easy to make.

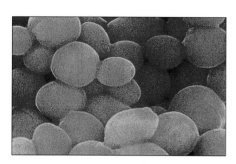

CANDIDA ALBICANS
The yeast Candida albicans *causes painful infections. To help prevent and control yeast infections, eat two or three 8-oz containers of yogurt a day. Yogurt can also be applied directly to the infected area to bring relief from itching and to help cure the condition.*

VERSATILE FOOD
Because the milk sugar (lactose) has been broken down by bacteria, yogurt is more easily digested than milk. This makes it an excellent food for newly weaned babies, elderly people, and people suffering from lactose intolerance.

Yogurt is known for both its healing properties and as a nutritional boon. It is an excellent source of milk nutrients, such as protein, calcium, potassium, and riboflavin. Many medical practitioners recommend yogurt to postmenopausal women, because it is such a rich and easily digested source of calcium, which maintains bone density and helps to prevent the brittle-bone disease osteoporosis.

INFECTION-FIGHTING PROPERTIES

Research conducted by Dr. Eileen Hilton at the Long Island Jewish Medical Center, New York, has substantiated the claim that yogurt is an effective treatment for vaginal yeast infections such as thrush. A group of women with a history of chronic yeast infections agreed to eat an 8-ounce portion of yogurt containing the *Lactobacillus acidophilus* culture each day for six months. As a result, they suffered far fewer yeast infections than a control group who did not eat yogurt.

Research conducted by Dr. George M. Halpern at the University of California School of Medicine at Davis indicated that yogurt may also boost the immune system. People in the study who ate two 8-ounce containers of yogurt containing *Lactobacillus bulgaricus* and *Streptococcus thermophilus* each day for four months had significantly higher blood levels of gamma-interferon, one of the body's infection-fighting substances. Further studies by Dr. Halpern found that regularly consuming yogurt also cut the chances of catching a cold by about 25 percent and reduced the symptoms of hay fever by a similar amount. Yogurt is also thought to increase the activity of NK (natural killer) cells in the body, which are known to attack viruses.

Does only "live" yogurt work?
It was previously believed that only yogurt that contained live cultures of *L. bulgaricus*, *L. acidophilus*, and *S. thermophilus* had disease-fighting powers. But research by Dr. Joseph A. Scimeca at Kraft General Foods in the United States has shown that even yogurt that has had the majority of its live cultures killed by heating or freezing will substantially boost the immune system.

THRUSH

A very common infection, thrush is caused by the yeast *Candida albicans*. This yeast is always present in the body but certain conditions, as well as doses of antibiotics, can cause *C. albicans* to proliferate and produce the infection. Thrush usually affects the vagina but may also affect the mouth, throat, and anal area. Vaginal thrush produces a thick white or yellow discharge and intense irritation; oral thrush causes white patches in the mouth; and anal thrush is associated with a rash and irritation.

MAKING YOUR OWN YOGURT

Fresh yogurt is inexpensive and easy to make. All you need is a saucepan, a thermometer, a bowl, plastic wrap, and towel or a thermos, 2 cups of milk, preferably low-fat, and a tablespoon of unflavored yogurt.

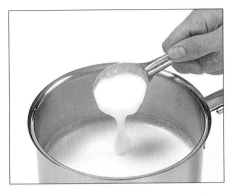

1 *Pour the milk into a saucepan and heat to the boiling point. Remove the pan from the heat and allow the milk to cool to 120°F. Add a tablespoon of plain yogurt to the milk as a starter and mix thoroughly.*

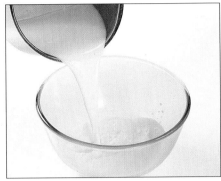

2 *Pour the mixture into a bowl and cover it with plastic wrap. Alternatively, pour the yogurt mixture into a thermos and then screw down the stopper.*

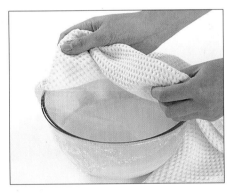

3 *If you are using a bowl, wrap it in a towel and put it in a warm place. Leave the mixture undisturbed until it thickens, usually after eight hours. Be careful not to let the mixture incubate for too long or it may start to separate.*

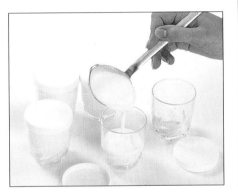

4 *Pour into cups and eat immediately or refrigerate. Yogurt will keep for up to five days. Save a tablespoon or two of your yogurt as a "starter" for the next batch. You may have to buy a fresh starter after making a few batches.*

TASTY VARIATIONS

If you want a yogurt with a creamier texture or a fresh tasty dessert, follow these suggestions.

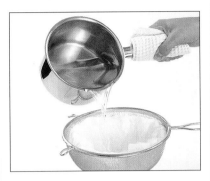

THICKER TEXTURE
To make a thick Greek-style yogurt, line a large colander or sieve with cheesecloth. Pour boiling water through the cloth to scald it. Place the colander or sieve over a bowl, pour in the yogurt, and let it drip overnight.

SWEETER TASTE
Add honey, chopped fruit, or unsweetened cooked fruit puree for sweetness and flavor after the yogurt has been made.

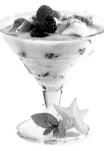

ICED DESSERT
Frozen yogurt made with low-fat milk provides a less fattening dessert than ice cream.

IDEAS FOR USING YOGURT

Yogurt is delicious eaten on its own, but combining it with other foods can provide a variety of nutritious snacks or meals. Choose low-fat or nonfat varieties.

▶ *Add yogurt to soups or casseroles to thicken and add creaminess. When cooking with yogurt, use a low heat; high temperatures can cause the mixture to curdle.*

▶ *Add lemon rind and paprika to yogurt to make a sauce for kebabs.*

▶ *Mix fresh herbs and garlic with yogurt to transform it into a delicious dip or dressing for salads.*

▶ *Use yogurt as a tasty topping for muesli or fruit desserts, potato salad, baked potatoes, and cold pasta dishes.*

▶ *Use yogurt instead of cream in cake fillings and frostings.*

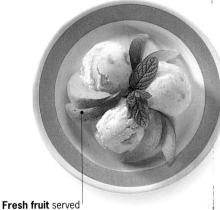

Fresh fruit served with yogurt adds fiber and vitamins.

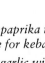

HARMFUL FOODS?

Not all foods that look and taste appealing are necessarily good for you. Some may cause health risks, while others could lead to allergic reactions.

Convenience and fast foods can be a satisfying and even necessary part of a busy lifestyle, but a diet overly reliant on such foods may lack variety, which is an important feature of a nutritionally balanced diet. Eaten too regularly, many packaged and fast foods may lead to health problems, due to their high-fat, high-salt, high-sugar, and low-fiber content Also, quite a number of such products contain additives that can trigger allergies or other conditions in susceptible people

WHAT'S IN A FAST MEAL?

A typical fast-food meal of a cheeseburger, french fries, and a milkshake contains around 1,000 calories, with 17 percent of the calories coming from protein, 39 percent from fat, and 44 percent from carbohydrate. Other such meals can be even worse. For instance, a British survey of fast foods turned up a sweet-and-sour dish from a Chinese take-out restaurant that contained a staggering 2,052 calories and 113 grams of fat (1,017 calories) per portion.

At least 20 percent of the fat in many packaged and fast foods is saturated, because it comes from meat, cheese, or highly saturated oils such as palm kernel or coconut. Too much saturated fat in the diet has been associated with increased levels of cholesterol in the blood, which increase the risk of heart disease.

When convenience foods are fried, the additional fat, even if unsaturated, can more than double the caloric value. Adolescents, who have high energy requirements, may easily burn up the extra calories, but in adults they quickly turn to body fat.

Sugar and fiber

Fat is not the only culprit in typical convenience and fast foods. Soft drinks, juices, and many crackers, as well as cookies, cakes, and other desserts, are often high in sugar. Particularly high are some of the "low-fat" baked goods.

Fiber, on the other hand, is conspicuous for its low levels in fast food. Diets with minimal fiber can cause constipation and may contribute to the development of colon cancer. The best fiber providers tend to be those foods not usually included on a fast-food menu—fruits, salads, and whole grains. For example, the typical buns for hamburgers and hot dogs are made with refined flour. Because fast-food outlets are not required by law to disclose what goes into their products, some consumers remain blissfully and perhaps dangerously unaware.

Sodium content

A typical hamburger from a fast-food eatery contains about 400 milligrams of sodium, and fried chicken can have more than 2,000 milligrams. These figures go even higher if you add pickle relish or cheese.

The biological need for sodium is only about 220 milligrams a day, the equivalent of one-tenth of a teaspoon of salt. The suggested maximum daily sodium intake, however, is higher—1,100 to 3,300 milligrams. But a steady diet of fast food, TV dinners, and canned products can easily exceed these amounts. Canned soups, especially, and beans and other vegetables tend to be quite high in sodium. Some manufacturers are offering no-salt or low-salt alternatives that make it easier for people who have sodium-restricted diets to meet their needs.

The possible harmful effects of excess salt are well documented, albeit with some controversy. Even though researchers have linked hypertension (high blood pressure) with a high sodium intake, there is no conclusive proof that sodium causes it. Eating less salt, however, does help to lower blood pressure in people who are salt sensitive.

FAST-FOOD MEALS

Fast-food meals are often popular with family members, but instead of buying takeout food, why not make your own quick meals. A homemade version of a hamburger and french fries can be just as tasty but have much less fat. Make the hamburgers with lean ground beef, then broil them. Slice scrubbed, unpeeled potatoes thinly, toss with a spoonful of olive oil, and bake in a single layer in a hot (400°F) oven until crisp and golden (about 45 minutes).

COMMERCIAL FAST-FOOD MEAL
A single meal of hamburger, fries, carbonated orange drink, and apple pie from a fast-food outlet will provide you with many of the essential nutrients. But the proportion of these nutrients may not be healthy.

A regular portion of fries
provides 210 calories; 3 g of protein; 26 g of carbohydrate; 10 g of fat, of which 1.5 g is saturated; 2 g of fiber; and 135 mg of sodium.

A medium-size carbonated soft drink
provides 210 calories; 55 g of carbohydrate (50 g of which are sugar); and 20 mg of sodium.

A 4-oz hamburger
provides 420 calories; 23 g of protein; 36 g of carbohydrate; 20 g of fat, of which 8 g is saturated; 2 g of fiber; and 690 mg of sodium.

An apple pie
provides 290 calories; 3 g of protein; 37 g of carbohydrate, of which 14 g is sugar; 15 g of fat, of which 3.5 g is saturated; 1 g of fiber; and 220 mg of sodium.

The pros and cons of salad bars

In a concession to the need for more healthful restaurant choices , the salad bar is now as ubiquitous as fast-food eateries. Many even provide complete meals, but their health benefits cannot be realized unless customers fill their plates with the right selections. If you are making a salad to complement a restaurant meal, select mainly raw vegetables and greens, and top with a low-calorie dressing. If you're creating an entire meal, choose a steamed or baked entrée, rice or potato, and vegetables, with perhaps a side of fruit. Items to avoid are croutons, bacon bits, creamy dressings, and salads made with mayonnaise.

FOOD ADDITIVES

As the popularity of processed foods increases, so does the concern about what manufacturers add to them. Preservatives are a common additive. They prevent the growth of dangerous microorganisms, such as bacteria, that can cause food poisoning, and extend a food's shelf life, making it less expensive and more widely available. Other kinds of additives are also used to make food more appealing in color, texture, and flavor.

All additives in foods sold in the United States must have been approved by the U.S. Food and Drug Administration and must be listed on the food labels.

Preservatives

Some of the traditional additives, such as nitrates, that are used to cure meats have been linked with cancer. However, they do prevent botulism, which is a deadly disease.

The benzoate preservatives, particularly calcium benzoate, are used for fruit preservation and are found in such products as fruit drinks and fruit pies. Some individuals may be sensitive or allergic to them.

Sulfites are used to preserve fruits, vegetables, and fish, as well as wine, beer, and cider. They should be avoided by asthmatics, as they may precipitate asthma attacks.

Chemical antioxidants are added to oils and fats to prevent their turning rancid. Two of these antioxidants, BHT and BHA, have caused concern and controversy. While some studies have indicated that BHT acts as a cancer promoter in rats, other studies have shown that it may actually guard against certain cancers and that rats fed BHT tend to live longer.

Colorings

Dyes are added to food to make it look more appealing. They have been highly criticized by consumers because, unlike preservatives, they do not increase the safety of food, only prettify it. Some colorings are natural, but a great number of the permitted colorings in North America are made in the laboratory. Of these, the most concern has been over the azo, or coal tar, dyes.

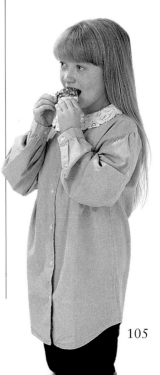

TREATING YOUR CHILD
Eating fast food is considered a treat by many children. It may be difficult to wean your children off such foods, but there are ways you can limit their intake. Satisfy a child's appetite with homemade "fun" foods such as pizza. Let her add the toppings of her choice.

Tartrazine, a yellow azo dye that is often used in children's drinks and candy, causes allergic reactions in some people. Asthmatics and persons who are sensitive to aspirin are more likely to be sensitive to tartrazine and other azo dyes. Such is the worldwide concern over coal tar food dyes that of the 19 permitted in the United Kingdom, only 5 are allowed in the United States. Tartrazine is banned in France and Belgium. The coal tar dye red dye number 2 is banned in the United States, whereas it is permitted in Canada, which bans red dye number 40. Norway has gone one step further by banning all artificial food colorings.

Flavorings

Thousands of different flavorings are added to processed foods. Some are natural; others are synthetic copies of natural substances.

THE PROS AND CONS OF ADDITIVES

The additives in a food or beverage must be clearly listed on the label, but the bewildering array of chemical names and numbers may be more confusing than helpful to the average consumer. The chart below describes various types of additives, the foods and drinks that usually contain them, and their helpful or harmful effects. Use the chart as a guide before shopping to help you make informed choices.

ADDITIVE	FOOD	PROS	CONS
PRESERVATIVES			
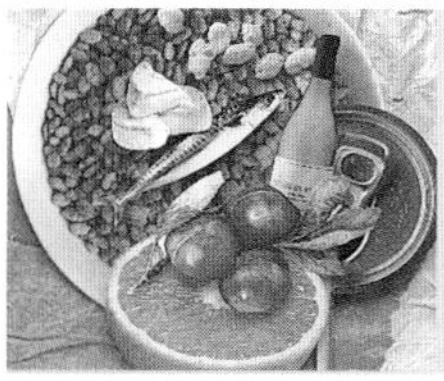 Nitrates, nitrites, BHT, BHA, benzoic acid, benzoates, ascorbic acid, sulfites.	Nitrates in vegetables; nitrites in cured meats; BHT and BHA in margarine and potato chips; benzoates in fruit drinks; sulfites in fruit juice, beer, wine, and cider.	Protect food from bacteria and fungi that cause food poisoning. Extend shelf life.	Nitrites are linked with cancer. Sulfites and benzoates can cause adverse reactions in asthmatics.
COLORINGS			
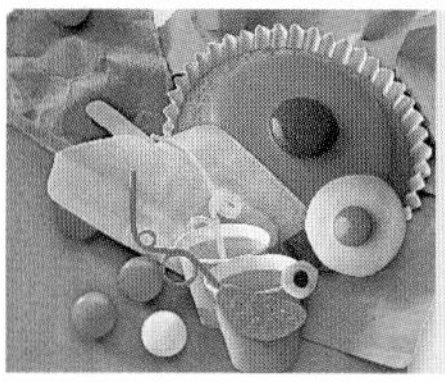 Natural substances, such as beta carotene, tartrazine and other azo, or coal tar, dyes.	Majority of processed foods. Tartrazine in children's drinks and candies.	Make food look more appetizing.	Azo dyes can cause allergic reaction in asthmatics.
FLAVOR ENHANCERS			
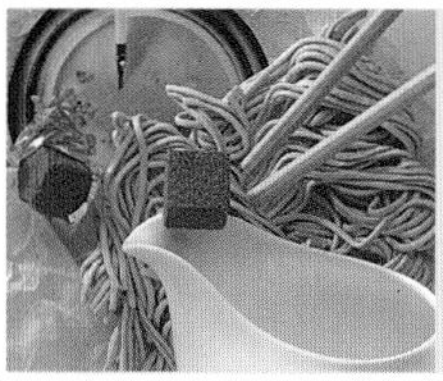 Monosodium glutamate, hydrolyzed vegetable protein.	Chinese food, gravy, soups, and snacks.	Enhance flavor.	Allegedly cause allergic reactions in some people.
STABILIZERS AND THICKENERS			
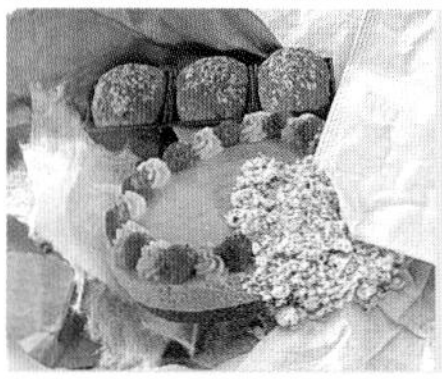 Gums, pectin, gelatin, cellulose, seaweeds.	Processed desserts, sauces, soups, and baked foods.	Improve consistency and texture.	Make food look more substantial than it really is. Large amounts can cause flatulence.
EMULSIFIERS			
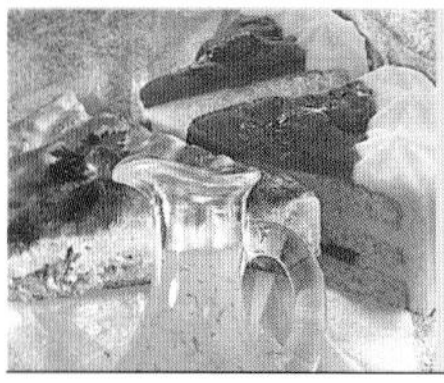 Lecithin, acacia.	Baked food, frozen puddings, and dressings.	Stop oil and water particles from separating.	Acacia causes allergic reactions in some people.

CHINESE RESTAURANT SYNDROME

In 1968, half an hour after beginning to eat a meal in a Chinese restaurant, an American physician suffered extreme discomfort. His head ached, and he felt a burning sensation in the back of his neck. The symptoms were traced to a high ingestion of monosodium glutamate (MSG), a flavor enhancer often used in Chinese cooking. The doctor later called this reaction to MSG the Chinese Restaurant Syndrome. Other people claim to have had similar experiences after eating Chinese food. There does not appear to be any lasting effect, but in 1980 a scientific review panel for the U. S. Food and Drug Administration advised that manufacturers limit the amount of MSG they add to foods and to label accordingly.

Neither natural flavorings nor their synthetic counterparts seem to cause problems. But monosodium glutamate (MSG), which, strictly speaking, is a flavor enhancer, may cause adverse reactions in some people. It is added to many savory foods, soups, and Chinese food—hence the nickname Chinese Restaurant Syndrome to describe the unpleasant reaction in sensitive people (see box above). MSG is present naturally in mushrooms, anchovies, and carrots.

Thickeners and emulsifiers

Thickening or bulking agents increase the amount of air or water a product can hold. Derived from natural substances like seaweed and vegetable celluloses, these are generally harmless. Large amounts of some thickeners may cause uncomfortable symptoms, such as abdominal distention.

Emulsifiers prevent the oil and water from separating in processed foods like mayonnaise and salad dressing. Lecithin, derived from soybean sources, is a popular emulsifier. It is natural and considered harmless in normal amounts. There have been reports, however, that the emulsifier acacia, found in frozen puddings and baked foods, causes an allergic reaction in some people.

Vitamins and minerals

Vitamins and/or minerals are added to some foods to enhance their nutritional value. Dairy processors usually add vitamin D to milk, as it aids in the absorbtion of calcium, and they sometimes add vitamin A to skim milk to compensate for the amount lost in removing cream. Cereal and bread manufacturers often fortify their products with niacin, riboflavin, thiamine, and iron to offset the losses from refining grains. The only danger

from such additions is that they can accumulate in the body to toxic levels if a person is taking vitamin supplements as well.

FOOD ALLERGIES AND INTOLERANCES

It is not only spoiled food and additives that can make people ill. Allergies or intolerances to many foods are widespread and seem to be increasing. A true food allergy, as opposed to an intolerance, provokes an abnormal response from the immune system. Compounds in usually harmless foods are mistaken for alien invaders by the immune system, which launches antibodies to combat the threat. The antibodies cause the release of inflammatory substances that can provoke a range of symptoms, from diarrhea and nausea to a potentially fatal swelling of the throat. Allergic symptoms usually manifest themselves in minutes, thus alerting susceptible people immediately to the problematic foods. Foods most likely to provoke reactions are milk, eggs, wheat, fish, shellfish, strawberries, nuts, and legumes, especially soybeans and peanuts. Unless the allergy disappears of its own accord, usually the only recourse is to cut the offending food out of the diet.

What is food intolerance?

True food allergies are rare, but food intolerances are fairly common. The adverse reactions can take hours or even days to set in because, unlike the case with true allergies, the immune system is not affected by food intolerance. Symptoms range from mild maladies like headaches, indigestion, depression, and diarrhea to chronic conditions such as rheumatoid arthritis, eczema, and irritable bowel syndrome.

Food diary

If you think you may be suffering an intolerance to something in your diet, keep a record of what you eat and whether there are any reactions afterward. This will help you to detect problem foods, if a pattern of illness emerges.

Note the date, time, and all the food and drink consumed. It often takes many hours for particular reactions to occur, so fill in your diary over several days or weeks.

According to a study by Dr. John O. Hunter of Addenbrookes Hospital in Cambridge, England, cereals, dairy products, products containing caffeine, yeast-based items, and citrus fruits are the most common sources of food intolerance. Wheat is the most troublesome food, upsetting 60 percent of trial subjects.

Enzyme deficiency

Two common food intolerances are known to be the result of an enzyme deficiency. Lactose intolerance is very common, especially among people of Asian, African, and Mediterranean descent, many of whom lack an enzyme in their intestine called lactase, without which the lactose (milk sugar) in milk and dairy products, such as butter and cheese, cannot be broken down. The resulting symptoms include stomach cramps, diarrhea, and gas. Similarly, a deficiency of the enzyme lipase in the intestine can result in problems with fats passing undigested into the lower part of the bowel.

Identifying the guilty foods

Food intolerance is often difficult to diagnose. Special clinics for treating food intolerance and allergy, which have proliferated in recent years, use a number of different methods to identify troublesome foods.

In patch tests, essences derived from suspect foods are placed on the skin to see if an allergic reaction takes place. However, a comparable reaction may not occur internally when the food is eaten. Another method, the elimination diet, banishes all but a few innocuous foods from the diet for a few days. Foods are then reintroduced one by one while any reactions are noted. But this method may not be entirely reliable because the patient's experience of previous adverse reactions to a particular food may trigger a psychosomatic reaction that mimics the allergic response.

Double-blind trials are probably the best way of identifying food reactions. Food suspected of causing a reaction is put into a capsule, while an identical capsule is filled with a nonreactive substance. Neither the doctor nor the patient knows which capsule contains the food. The patient then swallows one of the capsules and records whether it triggers a reaction. A true reaction will occur only when a capsule with food in it is swallowed. Providing that the offending food can be identified, cutting it out of the diet is an effective treatment.

Cutting out gluten

Once it is known that a food causes a reaction, the obvious treatment is to stop eating it. But, as many people who cannot eat wheat products have found, this is not always as simple as it sounds.

Anyone with an intolerance to wheat is actually reacting to gluten, a protein found not only in wheat but also in rye, oats, and barley. If gluten is eaten by people who are intolerant to it, they suffer from abdominal pain and diarrhea. Even the tiny amount of gluten in a communion wafer can trigger irritation in some individuals.

In rare cases, gluten intolerance is part of a disorder called celiac disease, in which a person is unable to absorb essential nutrients from the intestines. The condition, the result of a hereditary defect, may lead to other health problems, such as anemia. If you think that you or your child may suffer from gluten intolerance, it is essential to see

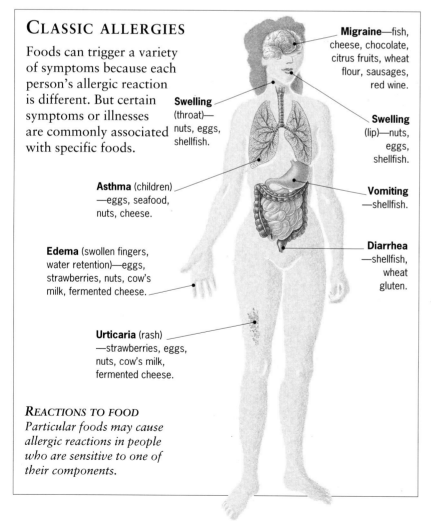

CLASSIC ALLERGIES

Foods can trigger a variety of symptoms because each person's allergic reaction is different. But certain symptoms or illnesses are commonly associated with specific foods.

Swelling (throat)—nuts, eggs, shellfish.

Asthma (children) —eggs, seafood, nuts, cheese.

Edema (swollen fingers, water retention)—eggs, strawberries, nuts, cow's milk, fermented cheese.

Urticaria (rash) —strawberries, eggs, nuts, cow's milk, fermented cheese.

Migraine—fish, cheese, chocolate, citrus fruits, wheat flour, sausages, red wine.

Swelling (lip)—nuts, eggs, shellfish.

Vomiting —shellfish.

Diarrhea —shellfish, wheat gluten.

REACTIONS TO FOOD
Particular foods may cause allergic reactions in people who are sensitive to one of their components.

a doctor for diagnosis. The disorder cannot be cured, but elimination of gluten from the diet will help to restore normal health.

Identifying an obvious gluten-containing food such as bread is fairly straightforward. Cakes, cookies, granola, oatmeal, and pasta are also easy to single out. But problems arise with processed and ready-made foods. Wheat flour is often used as a thickener and is found in all sorts of products. Food labels can help but may not be foolproof. If any of the following items are listed, it can mean that there is gluten in the food: edible starch, mixed grain, whole grain, multi-grain, vegetable protein, food starch, rusk, thickener, and bran.

Faced with such a minefield, sufferers often settle for a diet without any processed foods. Dried beans, nuts, rice, and corn are used as staples. Eggs, beans, fish, milk, cheese, and meat provide protein. Vitamins can be obtained from fruits and vegetables. And variety can come in the form of butter, cream, herbs, honey, jam, salt, spices, sugars, and yogurt.

THE CHOLESTEROL CONNECTION
A high level of cholesterol in the blood is associated with a thickening of the arteries (atherosclerosis), hypertension, and heart disease. But reducing your cholesterol level need not mean unreasonably restricting your diet. Eating the right foods can encourage your body to shed excess cholesterol.

Reducing the amount of high-cholesterol foods like eggs, cheese, and meat in your diet does help to reduce the body's cholesterol level, but not enough, because the body makes its own cholesterol. This wax-like substance is essential for many vital processes such as producing new cells and certain hormones. Depending on your body weight, from 800 to 1,000 milligrams of cholesterol are produced each day in the liver. The body also operates a balancing mechanism: When extra cholesterol enters the system through diet, less is produced in the body and more is excreted. Thus in most people, the cholesterol level stays much the same all the time.

Is cholesterol harmful?
Although there is little doubt about the relationship between high serum, or blood, cholesterol levels and heart disease, questions arise about the role of dietary cholesterol in heart disease. Some scientists maintain that a diet high in saturated fat (which reduces the body's ability to clear cholesterol) is the main cause of high blood cholesterol levels, not foods rich in cholesterol itself, like eggs, cheese, and meat.

Children and food reactions
Genuine food allergies are far less common than is generally believed, and although some are dangerous, most food reactions tend to be mild and disappear with age. The more serious ones can affect the absorption of nutrients, leading sometimes to dangerous weight loss or stunted growth. One such condition is celiac disease. About one in 2,000 children suffers from an intolerance to gluten, found in oats, barley, rye, and wheat, which leads to an inflammation of the small bowel. A gluten-free diet is the only way to relieve the symptoms. Other common food reactions are to milk, eggs, soy, chocolate, tea, and corn.

WHAT TRIGGERS AN ALLERGIC REACTION?

When an allergen enters a body, it causes a reaction in mast cells, defense cells commonly found in the linings of the stomach and lungs. These mast cells are covered with specific immunoglobin E (IgE) molecules, produced by the immune system the previous time the allergen invaded. Now the IgE and allergen molecules combine.

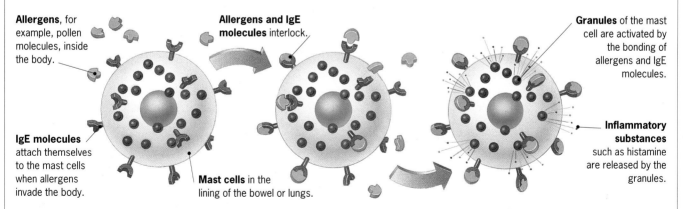

Allergens, for example, pollen molecules, inside the body.

Allergens and IgE molecules interlock.

Granules of the mast cell are activated by the bonding of allergens and IgE molecules.

IgE molecules attach themselves to the mast cells when allergens invade the body.

Mast cells in the lining of the bowel or lungs.

Inflammatory substances such as histamine are released by the granules.

SUSPECT MOLECULES
Allergen molecules enter the body via food, such as the protein in peanuts, or by inhalation, for example, of pollen.

INTERLOCKING
The allergen molecules bind with IgE molecules, which are attached to the mast cells as a line of defense.

PROVOKING A SYMPTOM
Mast-cell granules release inflammatory substances that cause such symptoms as sneezing or headache.

In fact, studies at Rockefeller University in New York revealed that an egg-rich diet raised the blood cholesterol levels in only two out of five people. And an analysis of various studies on cholesterol, made by Paul N. Hopkins of the University of Utah in Salt Lake City, concluded that in most people a high-cholesterol diet rarely raises blood cholesterol levels.

But not all research comes to the same conclusion. A study made by Dr. Richard Shekelle, professor of epidemiology at the University of Texas in Houston, found that people who ate high levels of cholesterol-rich foods lived an average of three fewer years than those who ate low-cholesterol diets. He also found evidence that a high intake of dietary cholesterol could stimulate the blood to make more clots and thus promote heart disease.

Because of the body's balancing act, scientists have suggested a new way of tackling the cholesterol problem. Rather than simply restricting high-cholesterol foods, individuals should eat foods that increase the "good" cholesterol, encourage the body to lose cholesterol, and protect cholesterol from oxidation (see page 111).

WHAT IS "GOOD" CHOLESTEROL?

Cholesterol is categorized according to the type of lipoprotein on which it is carried through the bloodstream. The "good" kind is HDL (high-density lipoprotein), and the "bad" is LDL (low-density lipoprotein). High levels of LDLs are associated with clogging of the arteries, which causes heart disease. High levels of HDLs, on the other hand, help to prevent this from happening because they collect and remove excess cholesterol from tissues and serum. Certain foods can reduce LDLs and boost HDLs, thus protecting against heart disease.

In 23 out of 25 studies, oat bran has been shown to reduce overall levels of cholesterol. More interesting, though, is the fact that oat bran may reduce detrimental LDLs and boost beneficial HDLs. Researchers have claimed that oatmeal boosts HDLs by about 15 percent after two or three months. Oat bran's weapon against cholesterol is believed to be high levels of beta glucans, a soluble fiber (see page 46).

Foods that boost HDLs

Research conducted by Dr. James Anderson of the University of Kentucky College of Medicine revealed that just one cup a day of a food rich in soluble fiber—like oat bran—reduces LDLs by about 20 percent and boosts HDLs by 9 percent in the long term. The pectin in fresh vegetables and fruits also provides soluble fiber; good choices include brussels sprouts, parsnips, okra, peas, and broccoli, which are valuable sources, as are oranges, apricots, and mangoes.

Grapeseed oil may also boost HDL cholesterol. When David T. Nash at the State

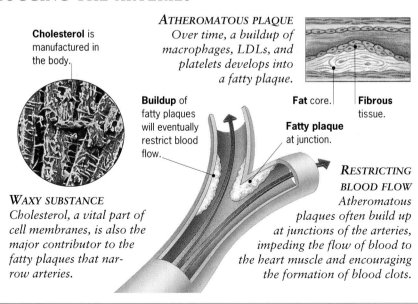

CLOGGING THE ARTERIES

Heart disease is caused by reduced blood flow to the heart muscle because of narrowed arteries (atherosclerosis). High levels of LDLs penetrate the inner lining of the artery and become trapped.

Macrophages (white blood cells that normally scavenge and inactivate or kill infectious and foreign agents) swallow the LDLs and combine with the platelets (blood cells that assist in blood coagulation) to form plaques. Over the years these plaques slowly build up, narrowing and possibly blocking the artery, making clotting more likely to occur. This will cause complete blockage of the artery.

Cholesterol is manufactured in the body.

ATHEROMATOUS PLAQUE
Over time, a buildup of macrophages, LDLs, and platelets develops into a fatty plaque.

Buildup of fatty plaques will eventually restrict blood flow.

Fat core.

Fibrous tissue.

Fatty plaque at junction.

WAXY SUBSTANCE
Cholesterol, a vital part of cell membranes, is also the major contributor to the fatty plaques that narrow arteries.

RESTRICTING BLOOD FLOW
Atheromatous plaques often build up at junctions of the arteries, impeding the flow of blood to the heart muscle and encouraging the formation of blood clots.

University of New York Health Science Center in Syracuse gave grapeseed oil to 23 men and women with low levels of the beneficial HDLs, he found "their HDLs went up on average by 14 percent. Some did not respond but the HDLs did go up in more than half of them." Nash concluded that the people with the highest HDLs (those over the age of 55) were the least likely to benefit from the oil. However, this study has not been substantiated by others.

The benefits of alcohol

Wine, especially red wine, is also credited with raising the levels of HDLs. But even beer can do so. A study in the United Kingdom found that a moderate intake of beer—a glass or two a day—boosted HDLs by about 7 percent. A similar study had even better results; HDLs were boosted by 17 percent with a daily intake of 1.3 ounces.

Cooking oil and cholesterol

Most vegetable oils consist primarily of unsaturated fats, which help to lower overall levels of cholesterol. The oils that are highest in polyunsaturated fats—corn and safflower—have been shown in tests to lower overall cholesterol levels by as much as 10 percent. But the oils higher in the monunsaturated fats—canola and olive—seem to be more discriminating, lowering mainly the LDL (bad cholesterol) level and raising the level of HDLs.

How does olive oil help?

In addition to lowering overall cholesterol and boosting HDLs, olive oil may protect the heart in yet a third way. This has to do with the manner in which LDLs clog the arteries. The theory is that rogue molecules called free radicals collide with the LDLs, becoming fixed to them via an oxygen link. These oxidized LDLs are then swallowed by macrophages, white blood cells that normally protect against foreign bodies, including infectious fungi, bacteria, and viruses. The macrophages then join with platelets, making enlarged cells that go on to form fatty plaques that build up over many years, eventually restricting blood flow.

Olive oil may protect against this oxidation in two ways. Whereas polyunsaturated fats are readily oxidized, the monounsaturated fat in olive oil is less prone to damage from oxidation. Second, olive oil contains antioxidants that are thought to mop up free radicals, thus reducing the likelihood of LDLs coming under attack in the first place. The role of antioxidants in preventing disease appears to be increasingly influential.

However olive oil works, there is little doubt that it is effective. In Mediterranean countries such as Italy and Greece, where olive oil is the primary cooking oil, the rates of heart disease are significantly lower than in countries like the United States—despite similar intakes of fat and cholesterol in the diet (see page 114).

Cholesterol levels

In general, cholesterol levels should be maintained at under 200 milligrams per deciliter (mg/dl) of blood. (Recent studies showed that people past age 70 can have a higher level without increased health risks. This is still being investigated.) If your level is over 239 mg/dl, your doctor will measure the amount of HDLs and LDLs that are present. Their relative levels are an important factor in determining your risk. Premenopausal women tend to have higher levels of HDLs than men, because estrogen raises their HDL level. At least 45 mg/dl or above of HDLs offers protection against heart disease. The risk of heart disease increases when the level of HDLs is 35 mg/dl or lower. A dangerous level of LDLs is 160 mg/dl or more; under 130 mg/dl is desirable.

"GOOD"-CHOLESTEROL DIET

Eating foods that increase "good" cholesterol (HDL) and reduce overall cholesterol levels does not have to mean a sudden and dramatic change to your diet. Introduce the following measures gradually and then make them a regular part of an overall healthful eating plan.

▶ *Boost your intake of lean foods, such as fish and skim milk, while reducing consumption of saturated fats, such as butter.*

▶ *Eat a bowl of oatmeal for breakfast.*

▶ *Eat plenty of fresh fruits and vegetables, at least five servings per day.*

▶ *A moderate amount of alcohol can boost HDL levels. But too much alcohol can have the opposite effect.*

▶ *Increase your intake of dried beans, grapefruit, bran, garlic, onions, apples, wholegrain cereals, soy products, almonds, and walnuts—all may lower overall cholesterol levels.*

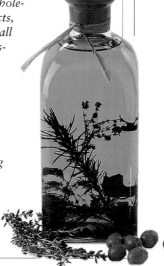

LIFE-ENHANCING OIL
Use polyunsaturated fats like corn oil and sunflower oil for cooking or in salads. Better still, use olive or canola oils, which are high in monounsaturates.

FRESH OR STALE?

Because eggs are highly perishable, special care should be taken to prevent illness. Follow these precautions when choosing and storing eggs.

▶ *Always check the "sell-by" date on carton.*

▶ *Do not use cracked eggs, because they may contain bacteria.*

▶ *Store eggs pointed end down.*

▶ *Store eggs in their carton inside the refrigerator. Put leftover raw eggs in a tightly covered container in the refrigerator. They will keep for two days, egg whites for up to two weeks.*

▶ *Eat egg dishes immediately or refrigerate them. It is vital that people "at risk" from salmonella—babies, children, pregnant women, and elderly people—should not eat raw eggs at all.*

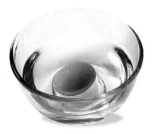

TOO OLD TO USE
To test the freshness of an egg, put it in a bowl of water. Fresh eggs sink to the bottom, while stale eggs float, rounded end up, to the top because the size of the air pocket increases with age.

THE TRUTH ABOUT EGGS

Inexpensive, nutritious, and versatile—what could be better than an egg? But scares about cholesterol and salmonella have tarnished its reputation in recent years.

Nutritionally, eggs have much to recommend them. The average egg contains about 6 grams of high-quality protein, which is roughly 15 percent of an adult's daily requirement. An egg also supplies modest amounts of important minerals, including phosphorus and calcium, and is a good source of vitamins B_2, B_{12}, D, and E. It is also low in calories (a large egg has 75 calories).

It is not surprising, then, that eggs were once considered an almost perfect food and a high consumption was recommended. But unfortunately, research into cholesterol showed that, at about 213 milligrams per large egg, cholesterol content is high. Since the suggested daily intake of cholesterol is only 300 milligrams, it is easy to see why dietary guidelines now recommend limiting egg intake to no more than four a week.

Some farmers in the United States have responded to people's worries over cholesterol by claiming to have produced a "low-cholesterol" egg through selective breeding and cholesterol-lowering feeds, such as fish oil. Even if the eggs are lower in cholesterol, say, 175 milligrams versus the usual 213, they still pack a cholesterol punch in excess of most other foods.

Using less egg yolk

Concerned consumers can reduce their cholesterol intake in better ways. All of an egg's cholesterol (and most of its nutrients) is found in the yolk. The white is mainly protein. In dishes like omelets, two whites can be substituted for one whole egg. In baking, a whole egg can be replaced with two egg whites, and two whole eggs can be replaced with one whole egg plus two or three whites. People who want to reduce cholesterol even more can use egg substitutes. These are frozen or powdered and usually contain very little cholesterol, as they are made from egg whites and monounsaturated oils. The main drawback is that egg substitutes also contain artificial additives.

Salmonella

The danger of salmonella poisoning from eggs has received massive publicity in recent years. Many hens harbor the disease-causing bacteria *Salmonella enteritidis*, which can be passed into the egg before the shell is formed. The result is a perfect-looking egg that is contaminated.

The salmonella bacteria can be destroyed by cooking. But some researchers claim that normal cooking temperatures are not high enough to do this. The bacteria could still survive in lightly cooked dishes such as soft-boiled or runny scrambled eggs or omelets. The raw egg in a traditional Caesar salad, and the uncooked egg whites in a frozen souffle definitely pose a risk.

Salmonella poisoning is especially dangerous for people whose ability to fight disease may be immature or impaired, including young children, the elderly, and people with immune-deficiency illnesses such as AIDS. Pregnant women, too, might pass the infection to their unborn babies. Those at risk should use an egg substitute or liquid pasteurized egg products, which are heat-treated to kill any pathogenic bacteria.

There is hope that salmonella may be eradicated in the not too distant future with a vaccine being developed for chickens.

NUTRIENTS IN EGGS

PRODUCT	CALORIES	PROTEIN (grams)	CARBOHYDRATE (grams)	FAT (grams)	CHOLESTEROL (milligrams)	SODIUM (milligrams)
Whole egg (1 large)	75	6.3	0.6	5.1	213	62.0
Egg yolk (1 large)	59	2.8	0.3	5.1	213	7.0
Egg white (1 large)	16	3.5	0.3	0	0	55.0
Egg substitute (1 oz)	25	3.6	0.1	0	0	53.0

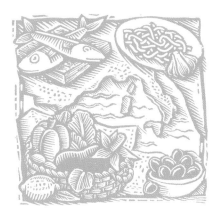

CHAPTER 8

THE BEST DIETS

Some populations are healthier than others, perhaps in part due to eating habits. Many people might benefit by including in their diets the nourishing, tasty foods eaten by people in the countries around the Mediterranean Sea, and in Japan and China. Conspicuously absent from these national cuisines are the large portions of fatty meats, rich dairy products, and highly refined and processed foods consumed by urban, industrialized Western peoples.

WHAT ARE THE BEST DIETS IN THE WORLD?

Living a long and healthy life depends on a variety of factors, and a well-balanced diet is one of the most vital. This can be demonstrated by observing the effects of certain national diets.

A flavor of the Mediterranean
Enhance your meals by experimenting with dried beans and legumes the Mediterranean way. Add chickpeas, lentils, or black-eyed peas to soups and stews. Serve salads of red kidney beans dressed with olive oil, lemon juice, crushed garlic, and fresh herbs. Or puree the beans with the same flavorings for dips and spreads.

FRUIT OF THE OLIVE TREE
Olives are harvested in many Mediterranean countries—Spain, Greece, Italy, Portugal, and Provence in the south of France. Like wine, the oils produced from olives have unique flavors and aromas that are dependent on the country of origin.

Every few years in the popular press, tales are told of remote, mountainous districts where residents live, hale and hearty, well past their 100th birthdays. The robust health and enviable energy of these individuals are attributed to some special ingredient in the local diet. The elixir may be live yogurt, wild garlic, or a particular sort of honey, but the claims made for it are sufficient to create a significant sales boom among health-conscious consumers.

Although no one has yet found the recipe for immortality, over half a century of scientific research has indicated that there are indeed parts of the world where the inhabitants enjoy lives that are far healthier than those of other regions. According to these studies, the traditional diets of China, Japan, and the countries on the shores of the Mediterranean Sea provide safeguards against a broad spectrum of debilitating and life-threatening illnesses, ranging from heart disease to a number of different cancers.

A WORLD OF DIFFERENCE
Within Europe itself, nutritionists have observed that a country's diet seems to become healthier in proportion to its proximity to the Mediterranean Sea. In the 1960's, for instance, a survey of food consumption patterns revealed that the average Spanish, Portuguese, and Italian citizen ate more than three times as many fresh fruits and vegetables in a year than his or her counterpart in Great Britain. And although diet may not be the only influence, it seems no coincidence that the two countries with the worst rates for cardiovascular disease are Scotland and Finland—both with very low intakes of fruits and vegetables.

It was only in the mid-20th century that links between food and health were first investigated extensively on a truly scientific basis. The statistics that began to accumulate revealed that even among affluent, developed nations with very similar standards of living, there were dramatic differences in the health of their populations.

Groundbreaking study
In the early 1950's an American nutritionist, Professor Ancel Keys, launched his groundbreaking "Seven Countries Study," a detailed scrutiny of the relationship between specific diseases and cultural variations in diet. Keys noted that only a very small proportion of people eating Mediterranean diets, like those of the Italians and Spanish, developed heart disease, in marked contrast to their U.S. counterparts, who were experiencing an increase in such cardiovascular complaints as hypertension, heart attacks, and strokes. Working with an international team, Keys established a close connection between dietary fat, blood cholesterol levels, and the incidence of heart disease.

For 10 years Keys and his colleagues studied men aged between 40 and 59 years who lived in rural areas on three different

RATES OF HEART DISEASE AROUND THE WORLD

Studies comparing the mortality rates of heart disease have shown marked contrasts between people eating different national diets. People whose diets are high in saturated fats but low in polyunsaturated fats as well as fruits and vegetables have a greater risk of developing heart disease than people with healthier diets.

COUNTRY	FEMALE	MALE
U.K.	198	498
Finland	140	489
Canada	102	383
Australia	143	374
U.S.A.	132	322
Germany	92	289
Greece	69	218
Italy	59	193
France	32	101
China	55	84
Japan	22	55

continents in seven different countries: the United States, Finland, the Netherlands, Italy, Yugoslavia, Greece, and Japan. A systematic comparison of these regional diets revealed that the men with higher blood cholesterol levels came from places where a lot of foods with large amounts of hard (saturated) fats from animal sources were eaten. These men also had a greater risk of dying of heart disease. But this higher death rate did not seem to be linked to the total amount of fat (saturated and unsaturated) in the diet or to the number of calories eaten.

THE PROTECTIVE OIL

Researchers found the incidence of heart disease to be substantially lower among those subjects eating diets rich in polyunsaturated fats, the fats found in vegetable oils, or in monounsaturated fats, the fats found in olive oil. The Mediterranean diet in particular, with its lavish use of olive oil, seemed to have a protective effect. Later research into the complicated subject of blood (serum) cholesterol has confirmed this view. The monounsaturated fats found in olive oil appear to lower the total quantity of cholesterol and the dangerous type of cholesterol (known as LDL) that clogs the arteries while at the same time increasing the amount of protective cholesterol (HDL) within the bloodstream, which clears excess cholesterol from the blood (see page 56).

More recent studies have reinforced the merits of the Mediterranean approach to food. The French National Institute for Health and Medical Research in Lyons set up a controlled experiment for two groups of heart-attack patients. In this study one set of subjects followed a Mediterranean-style diet using canola oil, which is rich in omega-3 fatty acids. The researchers used the other team as a control group and let them eat whatever they pleased.

After two years the researchers found that the death rate among the Mediterranean eaters was 70 percent lower compared with that among the controls. With such clear evidence they immediately abandoned the clinical trial and put the surviving members of the control group on the Mediterranean-style diet, which they were now convinced would improve many patients' longevity.

MODERN DISEASES

Every traditional diet is subject to change. In many parts of the world, in the second half of the 20th century, living standards have risen, science and technology have advanced dramatically, and people have moved in

The antioxidant effect
The bountiful supply of natural antioxidants, such as vitamins C and E and beta carotene, within the Mediterranean diet provides an armory of powerful defenses. These potent chemicals fight the destructive effects of free radicals and oxidants—rogue molecules that are formed in the body as a result of combining with oxygen and environmental and dietary contaminants (see page 94).

Lemons, oranges, tomatoes, red peppers, avocados, and parsley are all endowed with effective natural antioxidants.

MAKING YOUR OWN PASTA

Pasta is an extremely versatile food and a good source of carbohydrate, which provides a steady supply of energy. It is simple to make; the only ingredients you need are 2 lightly beaten eggs, 2 cups flour, and ¼ cup water. Let the noodles dry for an hour or two and then cook them in plenty of boiling, lightly salted water.

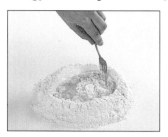

1 *Shape the flour into a mound on a smooth work surface. Make a well in the center and add the beaten eggs and water. Draw the flour into the liquid.*

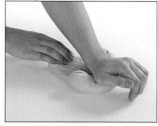

2 *Hold the dough with one hand and use the heel of your other hand to push the dough away from you. Repeat, rotating the dough, until smooth.*

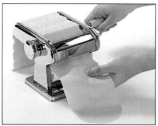

3 *Feed a lightly rolled-out portion of the dough through a pasta machine, taking care not to stretch or pull it as you guide it through.*

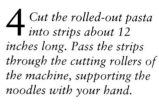

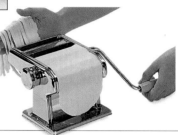

4 *Cut the rolled-out pasta into strips about 12 inches long. Pass the strips through the cutting rollers of the machine, supporting the noodles with your hand.*

The value of garlic

Garlic performs a number of healthy functions in the body. It is said to reduce the risk of heart disease by decreasing total blood cholesterol. Also, new research at Pennsylvania State University reveals that a compound in processed garlic, diallyl disulfide (DADS), depresses the growth of colon, lung, and skin cancer cells.

*ENJOYING GARLIC RAW
Raw garlic's pungent flavor can be partially softened in a yogurt and herb dip.*

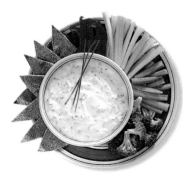

massive numbers from the countryside into ever-expanding cities. But this modernization has had its drawbacks. As the incidence of traditional infectious diseases decreased, people fell prey to what were, for them, a new set of plagues—illnesses linked with the lifestyles of the industrialized world.

For epidemiologists (scientists who deal with the causes and distribution of diseases affecting a population), the link between Westernization and the onset of certain diseases became easy to predict. As a country became more industrialized and more affluent, as its rural peasants turned into urban workers and their diets changed, the mortality rates from ailments such as heart disease and diabetes rose.

Ironically, it was these changes in eating habits and their demonstrated deleterious effect on the public's health that proved the value of the now-threatened traditional diets. In Greece, for instance, Professor Antonia Trichopoulou, of the National School of Public Health, monitored the effects on the population's well-being as people began to abandon the healthy diet that had sustained their ancestors for thousands of years. In 1989 she published a study showing that a dramatic rise in mortality rates from heart disease, diabetes, and cancers of the breast and colon had gone hand in hand with a 20-year increase in the consumption of animal fats and a corresponding decline in fruit and vegetable con-

sumption. Now Greece, like many other countries in the Mediterranean, is enthusiastically urging its citizens to return to the culinary traditions that nourished their great-grandparents.

A FEAST OF HEALTH

Anyone who takes pleasure in the vibrant colors and flavors of fresh fruits and vegetables, who savors the richness of olive oil, the tang of lemon juice, and the savory aromas of fresh herbs and garlic, will find no difficulty in embracing a Mediterranean-style diet. Much of it is familiar to lovers of good food: hearty vegetable and bean soups, a good helping of pasta lightly sauced with tomatoes and basil, a salad bowl full of crisp green leaves and topped with an olive oil dressing, and the freshest possible fish are all hallmarks of Mediterranean cuisine. A culinary voyage from Spain to southern France and Italy and on to Greece would reveal that, while different herbs or flavorings prevail, the principles remain the same.

These dishes are endowed with elements that promote good health. The dark-fleshed, oily fish beloved by Mediterranean diners—trout, mackerel, sardines, and many other varieties—are rich in omega-3 fatty acids. The unsaturated fats in these fish are also believed to have a strong protective effect on the heart and the entire vascular system, as well as to act as a deterrent against certain types of cancer and other diseases.

The Mediterranean lands abound with grains, vegetables, and fruits that thrive in their fertile soils. Incorporated into the diet, these foods provide dietary fiber—another essential ingredient for a truly healthy diet.

ORIENTAL DELIGHTS

Half a world away from the olive groves and vineyards of the Mediterranean shores, the traditional cooks of Japan and China have their own repertoire of life-enhancing, health-preserving foods, and culinary techniques. The international scientific community has shown particular interest in the Japanese diet, since the citizens of Japan enjoy the world's highest life expectancy and lowest incidence of heart disease and breast cancer. They do, however, suffer from a high rate of stomach cancer, which is thought to be linked to their heavy consumption of salty, pickled foods.

To a Japanese of traditional tastes, a meal centers upon complex carbohydrates, which are usually provided by several bowlfuls of rice. To vary the menu, Japanese cooks turn to several sorts of noodles derived from such starchy raw materials as wheat, mung beans, pea starch, and buckwheat, the latter sometimes blended with green tea, a rich source of catechins, which act as antioxidants and free radical scavengers (see page 94).

Dairy products, including whole cow's milk, cream, cheese, and butter, all of which are high in saturated fat, play almost no role in Japanese cooking. Meat is almost a condiment. It is shredded or cut into tiny pieces to flavor a dish of noodles or rice and is eaten in smaller quantities than in the West.

For protein Japanese cooks often rely on the highly nutritious soybean. In a process similar to cheese making, the beans are boiled down into a milk and the curds, known as tofu, are then formed into small blocks. Other vegetables are eaten raw or cooked only lightly by stir-frying, which preserves valuable nutrients.

Provisions from the sea

For most Japanese a major source of nourishment is the sea that surrounds their islands. Virtually every sea creature obtainable finds its way onto the Japanese table: squid and octopus, shellfish of all descriptions, oily-fleshed fish such as mackerel, bonito, tuna, and conger eel. As long as the fish is fresh and comes from unpolluted water, Japanese raw fish delicacies have all the virtues to delight a nutritionist's heart: they are high in protein, vitamins, and valuable minerals such as potassium, rich in omega-3 fatty acids, which help to protect against heart disease, and low in saturated

A gift of health from the sea

Coastal dwellers worldwide have always prized seaweed as a rich source of nutrients. These "sea vegetables" come in many varieties, from crinkly purplish dulse to deep green sheets of nori and dark strands of hiziki. Although high in sodium, they boast a wealth of amino acids, vitamin B12 (one of the few sources in the plant world), and minerals, including calcium, potassium, and iodine.

Nori seaweed

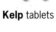

Kelp tablets

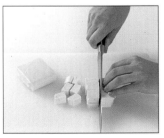

Fueru wakami

A TASTE OF THE OCEAN The marine flavor of seaweed adds an intriguing note to rice dishes and stir-fries. It is available dried in health food stores or—for the less adventurous—can be purchased in tablet form.

COOKING WITH TOFU

A delicate, silky substance, tofu, or bean curd, is one of the most versatile materials in the Japanese pantry: it can be steeped in an aromatic marinade and then broiled, stir-fried, or simmered with other ingredients in a broth. With only the subtlest flavor of its own, tofu readily takes on the taste of a sauce or any other ingredients that accompany it.

In addition to protein, tofu provides iron, calcium, and B vitamins. It contains little saturated fat and no cholesterol.

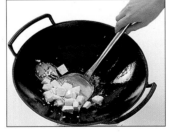

1 *Using a sharp knife, slice the block of tofu into several strips. Then, keeping the strips together, slice them into ½-inch cubes.*

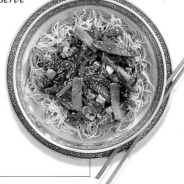

2 *Heat a little oil in a wok. Add some chopped garlic and cook for 30 seconds. Add the tofu in batches, stir until lightly browned, then remove.*

3 *Add vegetables and sauces. Cook for 2 minutes. Stir in tofu and stir-fry gently for 2 minutes. Serve with noodles.*

Tofu, lightly stir-fried with snow-peas, carrots, scallions, sweet peppers, and mushrooms and sprinkled with sesame seeds makes a delicious healthy meal.

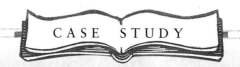

The Meat and Potatoes Man

People who have always eaten an American- or northern European-style diet, with large portions of meat and high-fat dairy products and limited use of fresh vegetables and grains, often find it difficult to adopt a lighter, healthier diet. Learning to cook Mediterranean style, however, offers many health benefits without too much effort.

Bill, aged 44, lives alone in a city apartment. Most of his dinners consist of a large helping of red meat, potatoes with butter, and canned carrots. His usual lunch is a tuna sandwich made with mayonnaise. When he works a late shift, he prepares a supper of eggs fried in butter, several strips of bacon, and thickly buttered toast. His father, who is in his early sixties, has recently suffered a stroke and has been told by his doctor that a lifelong diet high in saturated fats may well have been a contributing factor. Bill has read articles about the positive benefits of Mediterranean meals and now wants to try cooking them himself.

WHAT SHOULD BILL DO?

Bill should drastically cut down on his use of butter. He can still have a little on his toast but should start using vegetable oils for sautés or salad dressings. Bill also must eat much smaller quantities of meat, using it in combination with grains and fresh vegetables. He should look around his supermarket for types of fish that need little preparation, for example, salmon steaks and trout or mackerel fillets. Finally, Bill needs to increase his culinary repertoire. Newspapers and magazines often feature easy-to-prepare dishes, and there are plenty of cookbooks that contain Mediterranean recipes.

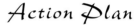

Action Plan

HEALTH
Visit a doctor to check blood cholesterol levels. Avoid whole-milk dairy products, which are high in saturated fat.

DIET
Buy vegetables that can be eaten raw in salads, such as tomatoes and carrots, or can be cooked easily, such as green beans.

EATING HABITS
Experiment with various foods that can be cooked quickly, such as foil-wrapped trout.

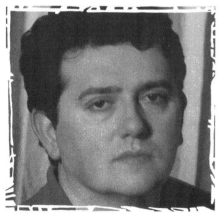

HEALTH
Eating foods such as butter and beef, which contain saturated fats, has the detrimental effect of elevating blood cholesterol levels.

DIET
Canned vegetables and fruits should be used only when fresh or frozen are not readily available. With the exception of canned beans and peas, a high percentage of vitamins is lost during canning.

EATING HABITS
Although frying foods may be quick, it is a very high-fat cooking method.

HOW THINGS TURN OUT FOR BILL

Although Bill's cholesterol levels were not dangerously high, his doctor told him to reduce his intake of saturated fats. Bill's supermarket stocks some fresh vegetables, such as spinach, that are ready to cook, which Bill now buys instead of canned varieties. He has also found a lighter, Mediterranean way of cooking eggs. One egg mixed with onions, peppers, and diced cooked ham makes the Italian omelet known as frittata. But he does occasionally have eggs and bacon when the pressure has been high at work.

fats. The sea is also a source of "vegetables" for the Japanese, who delight in the numerous varieties of seaweed that grow around their coastlines and use their salty intensity to season many dishes.

Flavors of the East

Many of the virtues of the Japanese diet can also be found in the culinary traditions of China, Japan's neighbor across the Yellow Sea. It is impossible to speak of a single Chinese cuisine: each region of this enormous and populous land has its own distinctive dishes, its own preferred ingredients and characteristic tastes. The intense, spicy-hot flavors of the western region of Szechuan, for instance, stand in marked contrast to the delicately flavored and subtly blended seafood and vegetable combinations enjoyed by the Cantonese of the southeast. But there are common traits. Like the Japanese, the Chinese derive the bulk of their nourishment from carbohydrates—grains such as rice and millet, and wheat made into noodles or into a variety of steamed breads, buns, and dumplings.

Some of the features that make a Chinese diet healthy are the result of thousands of years of scarcity and the need to conserve

THE ACCESSIBLE EAST

It is not necessary to live in the vicinity of an Asian market to adapt the healthful cooking ingredients of those from China, Thailand, or Japan. The classic elements of Far Eastern cuisine—gingerroot, fresh garlic, bean sprouts, scallions, leafy green vegetables, and traditional condiments such as soy and chili and black bean sauces of different intensities—can be found in most supermarkets.

INGREDIENTS
Many Asian foods are familiar to Western cooks.

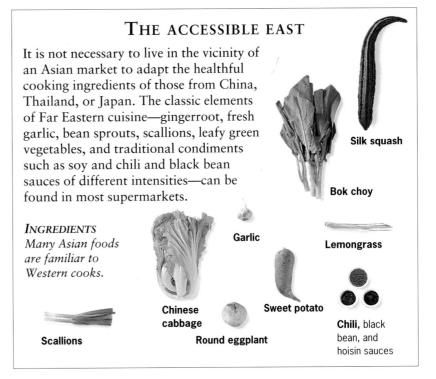

Silk squash

Bok choy

Garlic

Lemongrass

Sweet potato

Chili, black bean, and hoisin sauces

Chinese cabbage

Round eggplant

Scallions

precious resources. The classic Chinese technique of stir-frying—the use of a small amount of oil, heated in a round-bottomed vessel called a wok, for high-speed cooking of thinly sliced or diced ingredients—is a good example. This method emerged, in part, from a need to conserve fuel in a land that had little wood or other combustible energy sources to burn. But the benefits go beyond economy and ecology: the vegetable oils used in stir-frying are mainly polyunsaturated, and the cooking itself is so swift that few nutrients are lost.

Steaming is another energy-efficient and healthful Chinese cooking method. Stackable, flat-bottomed, openweave baskets of bamboo, piled up one on top of another, are placed on top of a vessel filled with boiling liquid. As the steam rises, it cooks the foods on each tier as it passes through; since no liquid touches the food, very few nutrients leach into the water.

One common element of these diets is their ingenious use of a few simple ingredients. Combining small amounts of meat or fish with lightly cooked vegetables and plentiful amounts of rice or noodles, and adding distinctive herbs and spices, makes a little protein go a long way. The results bring together the delights and virtues of the Far Eastern diet: fresh flavors, health-giving ingredients, and very little fat.

EQUIPMENT
Asian cooking techniques require some pieces of equipment that differ from those used by Western cooks. But utensils such as steamers and woks are available in most cookware shops.

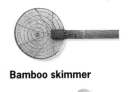

Bamboo skimmer

Wooden rice paddle

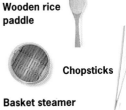

Chopsticks

Basket steamer

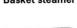

Cleaver

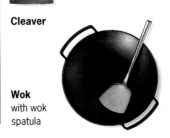

Wok
with wok spatula

EATING FISH RAW

For Japanese cooks the freshness of fish is paramount. No fishmonger in the world faces a fussier set of customers, especially when the seafood is destined to be served in the celebrated assemblages of raw fish known as sushi and sashimi.

EXOTIC TASTES
Sushi is a carefully crafted parcel of fish, roe, or vegetables and lightly vinegared rice. Sashimi is an array of thinly sliced seafood, sometimes served over rice.

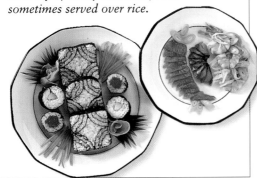

MEETING YOUR FAMILY'S NEEDS

At each stage of life, the calories and nutrients required are different. Lifestyle, activities, gender, and certain medical conditions also affect nutritional needs.

An energetic toddler, a teenager experiencing growth spurts, a pregnant woman, an adult who spends several hours a day sitting at a desk, another adult who earns a living out of doors in a physically demanding trade, a parent who goes out to work and returns home to the second full-time job of running a home and a family, a woman going through menopause, an elderly retired person—all these people differ in the amounts and types of energy they expend and in the kinds of nutrients they require to keep themselves fit and healthy.

Active, healthy infants or small children need a high number of calories in their small intake of food. Consequently, infants and young children can eat a larger amount of calorie-rich fats than middle-aged adults. Because fats deliver, gram for gram, virtually twice as much energy as proteins or carbohydrates, they are a valuable source of calories for a young body, which requires an enormous amount of energy to grow and thrive. Five- to six-year-old children need at least 1,710 calories a day. Most nutritionists also believe that children, like adults, should avoid an excessive consumption of saturated fats in favor of monounsaturated or polyunsaturated fats.

A LIFETIME OF DIFFERENCES
During infancy and the years of early childhood, the body grows and develops at a phenomenal rate; virtually every intellectual

MEALS FOR A TODDLER

Although a toddler's food intake is small and may be limited to a few foodstuffs, he or she requires, per body size, more nutrients than the rest of the family.

Whole-wheat cereal with whole milk provides fiber and calcium.

Ground lean meat is a rich source of iron.

Mashed potato with cheese provides carbohydrate, protein, and fat.

Bananas supply fiber; cottage cheese is protein rich.

Eggs are a valuable source of quality protein but must always be well cooked. Serve on a bed of salad, which provides vitamin C.

FUSSY EATERS
Toddlers can be very picky eaters. Make foods more appealing by presenting them in interesting shapes and colors.

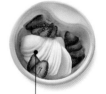

Pears and strawberries offer fiber and vitamin C.

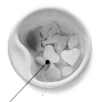

Cheddar cheese is a concentrated source of protein, fat, and calcium.

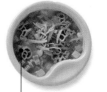

Pasta and vegetable soup is a good source of complex carbohydrates.

Yogurt and fruit milkshake supplies protein, fat, calcium, and vitamins.

and physical faculty is being stretched and exercised. And as anyone who has ever been surrounded by a roomful of preschoolers knows, toddlers are capable of sustaining a fierce and furious level of physical activity, never walking when they can run, rarely speaking when they can shout, and moving frantically from one new source of stimulation to another.

The middle-aged male, however, no matter how active his lifestyle, no longer needs a hefty intake of calories for growth. If he does find himself growing at all, it is inevitably an unwelcome expansion around his waistline. And apart from the relatively small percentage of the population working in highly demanding physical jobs, as a farm hand or as a laborer on a building site, for example, many middle-aged men are engaged in occupations requiring little expenditure of physical energy. They sit while they travel to work—in a car or on a train or a plane—and are likely to remain seated throughout much of the working day and possibly for most of their leisure hours.

For this reason, the calorie intake that turns the child into a powerhouse of healthy growth becomes, in a middle-aged man or postmenopausal woman, a dangerous cargo of excess nutritional baggage. It increases their risk of heart disease, hypertension, and stroke and imposes an unhealthy burden on the circulatory system. Conscientious efforts to eat a balanced diet and maintain a regular routine of physical exercise are essential to help keep adults fit and healthy. But they will never be able to consume the same generous helpings of calories, taken as a percentage of body size, that are eaten and burned up every day by an exuberant, healthy five-year-old child.

A vital role

Faced with the different nutritional needs of every member of the family, health-conscious cooks may well feel as if they have been thrust under the spotlight in a circus ring to perform a juggling act involving several different meals consisting of different ingredients and served at different times. But the task is not as daunting as it seems at first glance. The essential thing to remember is that everyone, whatever age, gender, or lifestyle, will benefit from a balanced, varied diet that is well supplied with complex carbohydrates, especially whole grains and

MEALS FOR A TEENAGER

Many adolescents eat a high-fat diet, which provides them with plenty of energy. But like everybody else, they need to have a good intake of fresh fruits and vegetables.

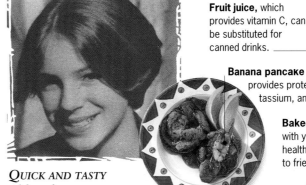

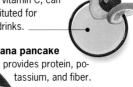

QUICK AND TASTY
Although many teenagers enjoy the taste and convenience of fast foods, some nutritious dishes can be just as easy to make.

Fruit juice, which provides vitamin C, can be substituted for canned drinks.

Banana pancake provides protein, potassium, and fiber.

Baked potato skins with yogurt dip make a healthier alternative to fries.

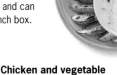

Vegetable frittata is simple to make and can be packed in a lunch box.

Fruit ices are fat-free and rich in vitamin C.

Chicken and vegetable stir-fry is an excellent source of protein, vitamins, and minerals.

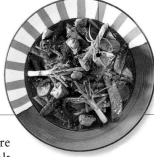

fresh vegetables and fruit. These foods are healthy because they are moderate in salt and sugar content, low in saturated fats, and good sources of vitamins and minerals.

Some family members may need special foods to fill particular nutritional needs; others will do better simply to skip particular foods or cut down and eat a little less than habit dictates. But no matter what the variations in personal requirements or preferences, it is not necessary to transform your kitchen into a full-service restaurant, providing completely different menus to each person in the household. Simply knowing the people you live with and taking a few minutes to consider their different needs are the most important steps you can take.

continued on page 124

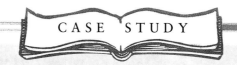
A Multigenerational Family

Providing healthy meals for a family that spans three generations is a considerable challenge, especially when individual members of that family have different lifestyles, special health concerns, and varying likes and dislikes. If the person feeding the family is juggling this responsibility with the demands of a job, the task can be even more daunting.

Anne Martin, who is 38 years old, and her husband, Peter, who is 46, have three children: baby Jess, who has just celebrated her first birthday, 8½-year-old David, and Erica, aged 14. The family also includes Anne's 72-year-old father, Tom, who has been living with the Martin family for three years, since the death of Anne's mother.

Peter commutes by train to his job as office manager for an insurance company. Anne works part-time as an admissions clerk at the local hospital, so little Jess spends Monday through Friday mornings at a day-care center. The two older children have a busy after-school schedule. David is a Cub Scout, and Erica has become the star sprinter for the girls' track team at her school. Anne worries that Peter, who spends so much of his day sitting down, is not getting enough exercise. The results of his sedentary lifestyle, coupled with the high-fat lunches in the office cafeteria, are beginning to show around his waistline. Working in a hospital, she has seen men even younger than her husband suffering from heart problems and heart attacks. She also is concerned about her father, who,

although he seems in reasonably good health for his age, suffers from constipation. And Anne worries about her children's nutrition. She was alarmed to discover, when she took the baby for her last checkup, that Jess is slightly underweight for her age. Anne also knows that a lively eight-year-old and an adolescent athlete need a well-balanced diet that will give them plenty of energy. Steering them away from junk food sometimes seems like a losing battle, especially with a young son who regards most fresh vegetables as a hostile alien life form.

CHILDREN
A study at the Children's Nutrition Center of the University of Texas found that 9- to 11-year-olds who missed breakfast performed less well on problem-solving exercises than those who regularly ate a morning meal.

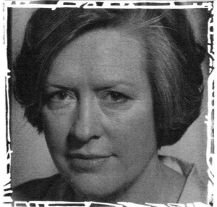

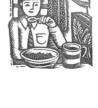

TEENAGERS
The enormous appetites of adolescents often go hand in hand with a social life that centers on the consumption of food notoriously high in fat or sugar: fast-food hamburgers, fries, ice cream, and soft drinks.

FAMILY MEALS
A high-fat diet, coupled with an inactive lifestyle, may lead to serious health problems, such as heart disease, in adults. But children often need the extra calories provided by fat.

TIME PRESSURES
Cooking with cereals, grains, and fresh vegetables is more labor intensive than simply slipping a couple of steaks or chops under the broiler or into the frying pan.

THE ELDERLY
Older people may suffer from a lack of iron, calcium, and certain vitamins. It is believed, for instance, that one of the side effects of aging is a decrease in the body's ability to retain vitamin C.

WHAT SHOULD ANNE DO?

Anne should begin by accepting that she is not the only person responsible for the entire family's well-being. Every member of the household, apart from tiny Jess, is capable of understanding the importance of eating healthfully and thinking about ways to improve his or her own diet. Rather than imposing rules that they will ignore, Anne should call a family conference to discuss the situation.

Instead of feeling guilty, Anne should start by thinking positively about the things she does right. For instance, she knows the importance of a good breakfast and makes the ingredients available to her family. She recognizes the need to cut down on the consumption of animal fats and simple carbohydrates, is aware of everyone's need for plenty of foods high in fiber, and appreciates the benefits of eating more fresh vegetables and fruit.

When the whole family is together, Anne should get them to suggest new, healthy recipes that they can try out over the next few weeks. She should also establish a rotation so that each person helps her to work out the shopping lists for the week.

To rouse the children's interest in food, Anne should ask the most artistic junior member of the household to decorate a scrapbook, large folder, or file box for storing healthfull eating ideas and recipes cut out of newspapers and magazines.

Action Plan

CHILDREN
For breakfast, offer whole-grain, high-fiber cereals instead of sugary flakes with lower nutritional value. Provide fruit or fruit juice at breakfast. Granola bars could be substituted for cookies. Ask David what he would like to eat for lunch.

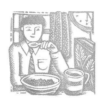

TEENAGERS
Stock up on the basics for healthy snacks: crunchy vegetables for eating raw, such as carrot and celery sticks, cucumbers, and cherry tomatoes; low- or reduced-fat dairy products, such as yogurt and low-fat cottage cheese, and healthy nibbles, such as raisins and unsalted nuts.

FAMILY MEALS
Encourage Peter to give up his cafeteria lunches and take a low-fat lunch to work at least four times a week. Cut down on the use of meat as a main ingredient and, apart from Jess, drink only low-fat milk. Offer Jess more whole-milk dairy products, such as yogurt flavored with fresh fruit.

TIME PRESSURES
Experiment with two time-saving "cook-in-advance" sessions every week to prepare large batches of vegetable soups and vegetable-rich stews—red-bean chili, for example. Such ready-to-eat meals will give the family a healthy and appealing alternative to fast-food meals.

THE ELDERLY
Make cooked fruit dishes and buy bananas, berries, and peaches for Grandfather Tom, who has false teeth and finds chewing crunchy fruits like apples difficult. Encourage him to visit the dentist to sort out denture problems. Urge him also to eat whole-grain breads and rolls.

HOW THINGS TURN OUT FOR ANNE

A few months into this new regimen, Anne feels she has the situation more under control. The baby is gaining more weight, and her husband, to Anne's great relief, is not, although she wishes he would exercise regularly. The switch to whole-grain breads has had an unexpected spin-off: Anne's father, convinced that no one makes bread the way he remembers it from his boyhood, has developed an interest in baking various breads himself and now spends happy hours providing the family's weekly bread supply. Anne wonders secretly if his improved temperament also has something to do with the digestive improvements caused by more fiber in his diet. The family's resolve to try as many new vegetable dishes and salads as possible has turned up a number of things that even her vegetable-hating son will eat, but Anne still finds herself fighting a losing battle in her efforts to ensure that David eats a healthy lunch. At school he tends to swap his apple for someone else's chocolate chip cookies. And no matter how many treats are in the refrigerator, the two older children are as likely as ever to contemplate the contents and complain that there is nothing in there to eat.

MEALS FOR A PREGNANT WOMAN

When expecting a baby, a woman needs extra protein and almost twice as much calcium as usual.

Cheese and ham omelet is high in protein and calcium.

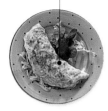

Granola with low-fat milk offers fiber and calcium.

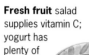

Fresh fruit salad supplies vitamin C; yogurt has plenty of calcium.

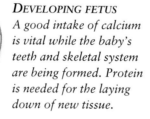

DEVELOPING FETUS
A good intake of calcium is vital while the baby's teeth and skeletal system are being formed. Protein is needed for the laying down of new tissue.

Chicken wrapped in cabbage with couscous is a good source of protein, vitamin C, and carbohydrate.

Raspberry tart supplies vitamin C, and the whole-wheat pastry offers fiber.

Greens provide folic acid, which helps to prevent birth defects.

Oranges are full of vitamin C, which aids the absorption of iron from carbohydrates and legumes.

The growing body

The basic principles of a healthy diet remain the same throughout life, but children, especially from infancy to age seven, have particular nutritional needs to support their development and promote good health. For example, even though whole milk is higher in saturated fat, nutritionists believe that babies and young children should drink it instead of skim milk to ensure they are not missing out on vital nutrients. The goal is to wean children onto low-fat milk, then skim milk by the age of seven.

Protein, too, because of its vital role in growth, is particularly important for the young. Adults and older children naturally produce all but eight of the amino acids that make up protein; they must obtain these missing elements from food. Babies and small children, however, lack another one or two of the essential amino acids, so they need to consume more high-quality protein, such as dairy products and poultry, to make up the shortfall. According to pediatric nutritionists, children between 1 and 3 years of age will need to eat 0.81 gram of protein per pound of their own body weight every day, while those between 7 and 10 years need only 0.55 gram. Adults, in contrast, require only 0.36 gram, less than half the amount recommended for the very young.

A pregnant woman or one who is breast-feeding a baby also has special needs, since what she eats has an effect on her child's

NUTRITION FOR ATHLETES

Athletes who make frequent and often punishing demands on their physical resources have special dietary needs beyond those of the ordinary person who exercises for good health.

For a long time it was believed that a large intake of protein was essential for athletic success—would-be Olympic champions and boxing contenders tradi-tionally fueled their training efforts with huge steaks for breakfast. While protein is important—especially for the repair of damaged tissue, such as the strains acquired on the sports field—contempo-rary nutritional thinking emphasizes the intake of unrefined complex carbohy-drates as a source of energy. The aspiring

track star is now more likely to eat huge helpings of whole-wheat pasta to stoke up with fuel for a forthcoming marathon.

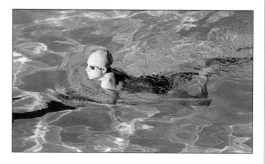

SUSTAINING ENERGY
To ensure a steady supply of energy during competition, athletes eat a variety of complex-carbohydrate foods the day before the event.

development. To help sustain the baby's growth and her own good health, she needs an iron-rich diet, with foods that are plentifully endowed with vitamin B$_6$ and folic acid—for example, spinach, cauliflower, broccoli, brussels sprouts, cabbage, and beans. And because the formation of the baby's bones and teeth will leach away her own supply of calcium, she needs to keep up her intake by drinking sufficient skim or low-fat milk and eating calcium-rich foods such as yogurt or sardines (with the bones).

The ravenous age

Teenagers' needs also differ from those of their elders. The constantly ravenous adolescent trawling the refrigerator is a familiar sight in many families. If based on healthy foods, the frequent snacks between meals that teenagers crave will help to supply the complex nutritional needs of a growing body passing through puberty. But the greatest challenge for the parents of a healthy adolescent is to ensure that the snack foods their son or daughter chooses will actually do some good. Processed products and greasy fast foods, high in saturated fat, salt, and sugar, are easy options for the teenager in a hurry, and may lead to poor nutritional habits that will be difficult to break and result in health problems, such as heart disease, in middle age.

For the teenager's parents, the consumption of frequent snacks could be a sure step on the road to obesity. Men of average height and frame need only approximately 2,550 calories a day, while women, because of a generally smaller build, are advised to consume a slightly lower intake—approximately 1,940 calories daily.

Slowing down

Nutritional requirements change sooner than one might think—at about the age of 35. Metabolism slows down, and people often become less physically active, so calorie intake should be scaled down accordingly, or exercise increased. A sedentary man in his sixties needs approximately 2,330 calories a day, while a woman in her sixties needs about 1,900 calories.

By a conscious adjustment of their dietary habits, such as cutting down their intake of foods high in fat, cholesterol, salt, and refined carbohydrates, and by eating plenty of foods high in fiber, adults can protect

themselves not only against becoming overweight but also against many of the illnesses that accompany aging. Current nutritional thinking, for example, suggests that all adults should consume an average of 18 grams of dietary fiber daily, in the form of fresh fruits, vegetables, and whole-grain cereals or whole-wheat breads; an elderly person might choose to increase this total to help combat constipation.

RESTRICTED DIETS

Whatever their ages, some family members may have dramatically different food preferences. Perhaps they are vegetarians who consume no meat, poultry, or fish but do eat dairy foods; or they may be vegans, who eat no animal foods at all, not even dairy products. These people have to obtain most or all of their protein, calcium, and B vitamins from plant sources, a task that calls for special planning to balance meals properly.

A family member who is trying to lose weight by following a calorie-controlled diet, depends not only on self-discipline but

MEALS FOR A MIDDLE-AGED PERSON

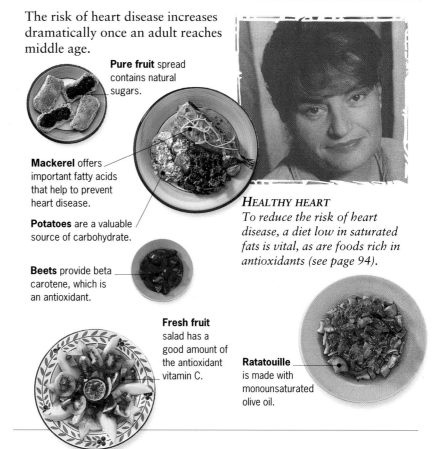

The risk of heart disease increases dramatically once an adult reaches middle age.

Pure fruit spread contains natural sugars.

Mackerel offers important fatty acids that help to prevent heart disease.

Potatoes are a valuable source of carbohydrate.

Beets provide beta carotene, which is an antioxidant.

Fresh fruit salad has a good amount of the antioxidant vitamin C.

HEALTHY HEART
To reduce the risk of heart disease, a diet low in saturated fats is vital, as are foods rich in antioxidants (see page 94).

Ratatouille is made with monounsaturated olive oil.

125

MEALS FOR AN ELDERLY PERSON

As a person grows older, extra fiber may be needed to prevent constipation. Some older people experience a diminished sense of taste and should guard against an overuse of salt.

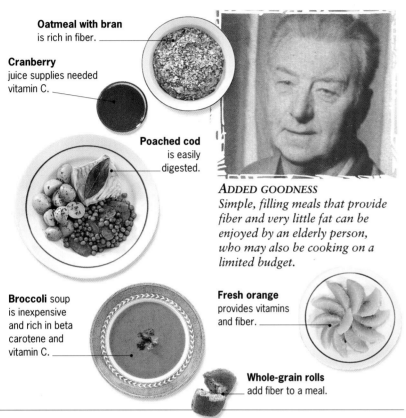

Oatmeal with bran
is rich in fiber.

Cranberry
juice supplies needed vitamin C.

Poached cod
is easily digested.

Broccoli soup
is inexpensive and rich in beta carotene and vitamin C.

Fresh orange
provides vitamins and fiber.

Whole-grain rolls
add fiber to a meal.

ADDED GOODNESS
Simple, filling meals that provide fiber and very little fat can be enjoyed by an elderly person, who may also be cooking on a limited budget.

also on the cooperation of anyone involved in shopping and cooking to ensure that meals contain low-calorie food choices and a minimum of fattening temptations.

Others may have dietary restrictions based on illness or high cholesterol. Certain medical conditions, such as diabetes or hypertension, require special consideration in planning and cooking meals and in the actual shopping for ingredients. Scrupulous label reading is necessary, for instance, to ensure that a hypertensive person—whose well-being may depend on a reduction of salt in the diet—is not being bombarded with the "hidden" salts found in so many processed and packaged foods. And a diabetic may have to not only restrict the intake of particular foods, such as sugar, but also pay special attention to the timing and composition of meals. Someone convalescing after serious illness, who may have a weakened immune system, also needs to receive the nutrients, such as proteins, vitamins, and minerals, that boost recovery and promote good health.

BURNING CALORIES

Even for people with no specific health concerns, differences in lifestyle have definite implications for diet. The caloric needs for a laborer doing heavy manual work far outstrip those of the deskbound. Since dietary

A SNACK AT HAND

HEALTHY INDULGENCE
Keep on hand a good supply of fruits, vegetables, nuts, seeds, and whole-wheat products to satisfy between-meal cravings.

The key to satisfying the needs and tastes of all family members can be found not only on the dinner table but also in the refrigerator and the cupboard.

The foods snack-hungry youngsters eat between meals are as important as those they consume around the family dinner table. Be sure always to have on hand a bowl laden with the most colorful array

of fruit that the season can provide; a selection of unsweetened whole-grain cereals, ready to eat with a little low-fat milk; a container, kept in the refrigerator, full of ready-to-eat raw vegetables, such as carrot sticks, cucumbers, and crisp wedges of red, green, and yellow peppers; and a supply of medium-fat or low-fat cheeses, such as cottage cheese or Neufchâtel.

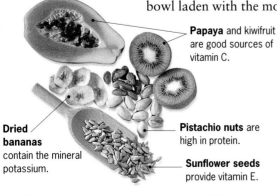

Papaya and kiwifruit
are good sources of vitamin C.

Dried bananas
contain the mineral potassium.

Pistachio nuts are
high in protein.

Sunflower seeds
provide vitamin E.

Carrots, tomatoes, and
red and green peppers are rich in the antioxidant beta carotene.

Low-fat cottage cheese is a
source of protein.

Whole-wheat crackers supply fiber.

Neufchâtel cheese
with salad in pita bread makes a nourishing high-fiber, low-fat snack.

fat contains twice the calories as the same weight of protein, only adults who burn up an enormous number of calories are likely to be able to sustain a high-fat diet without becoming overweight. For the average individual, nutritionists recommend that fat should provide no more than 30 percent of calorie intake, with a maximum of 10 percent of this fat consumption coming from saturated fats.

Nevertheless, anyone who has worked in a sedentary job, with set hours and a comparatively unchanging routine, knows how difficult it is to avoid the temptation to break up the routine of the working day with a quick foray to the nearest source of potato chips, chocolate bars, and soft drinks. But whenever you do succumb, you should adjust your calorie intake at home accordingly, since a can of cola or a chocolate bar can provide more than the maximum recommended simple-carbohydrate intake for an entire day. Alternatively, keep some healthy foods, such as dried fruits and whole-wheat crackers, in your bag or office drawer to help satisfy the urge for a snack.

PACKING HEALTH INTO A LUNCH BOX

The following tips will show you how to provide the members of your family with nourishing, tasty foods during their lunch breaks.

▶ *For sandwich fillings, use skinless chicken or turkey breast meat instead of fatty luncheon meats, ham, roast beef, or cheese.*

▶ *Moisten whole-grain bread with a smear of ketchup or mild mustard instead of butter or mayonnaise, and add crunch by lining the bread with crisp lettuce leaves and bell peppers.*

▶ *Reduce the fat in a tuna salad sandwich by using tuna packed in water and replacing regular mayonnaise with a low-fat type or low-fat yogurt and lemon juice.*

▶ *For a nutritious vegetarian sandwich spread, mix a small amount of peanut butter with a mashed banana.*

FEEDING A FAMILY

The best strategy for feeding a group of people with different needs is to plan meals around the common denominators and then add extras for those who need additional nutrients. A typical basic menu, for instance, might consist of whole-wheat pasta with a sauce made of onions, tomatoes, sweet peppers, mushrooms, and fresh herbs, accompanied by a leafy green salad, with a platter of fresh fruits and low-fat yogurt for dessert.

For someone who requires more protein —or is a determined meat eater—make the salad more substantial by adding lean cooked chicken or turkey. Fish, especially tuna or sardines, would add cholesterol-lowering omega-3 fatty acids as well.

A generous handful of bean sprouts, alfalfa sprouts, or radish sprouts or a sprinkling of wheat germ or sesame seeds will also boost protein.

Drinking a glass of low-fat milk with the meal will provide extra calcium for those who may need it, for example, a pregnant woman or a very young child. And both the pasta and the salad can be accompanied by small dishes of supplementary garnishes to be added as needed.

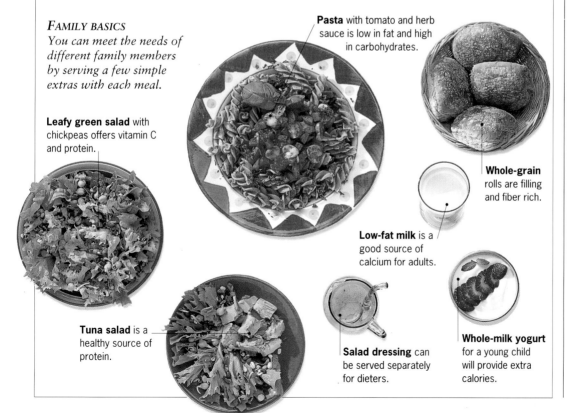

FAMILY BASICS
You can meet the needs of different family members by serving a few simple extras with each meal.

Leafy green salad with chickpeas offers vitamin C and protein.

Pasta with tomato and herb sauce is low in fat and high in carbohydrates.

Whole-grain rolls are filling and fiber rich.

Low-fat milk is a good source of calcium for adults.

Tuna salad is a healthy source of protein.

Salad dressing can be served separately for dieters.

Whole-milk yogurt for a young child will provide extra calories.

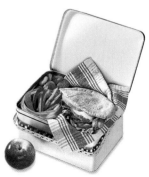

READY TO EAT
Tuck in easy-to-eat raw vegetables, fresh fruit, or such dried fruits as apricots or prunes, and sandwiches made with whole-wheat pita bread.

127

COOKING FOR YOUR CHILDREN

Children grow so fast, they need a higher proportion of nutrients in their diets than adults. They often prefer refined foods, however, and can sometimes be very picky eaters.

Children may refuse to eat for many reasons, few of which have to do with the food. Although your children may reject certain foods, if you offer a variety of nutritious foods that are cooked or presented in an appealing manner, you will find things they like that are good for them. If you are unsure about the nutritional content of your children's diet, contact your doctor for advice.

Problems with eating hot food

The flavor and texture of many foods change when they are cooked—and some children will balk at the difference. This change most often happens with vegetables. Children may gobble up raw carrots, for example, but ignore them cooked. If this is the case with your youngsters, let them eat cleaned raw vegetables. They generally have a higher vitamin and mineral content than cooked vegetables and are a good source of fiber. Introduce other cooked foods until you find some that your child likes.

Be patient and bear in mind that if your child is thriving—has an abundance of energy, sleeps well, is not underweight or overweight, and does not suffer from stomach cramps, constipation, or diarrhea—then he or she is developing well.

HEIGHT AND WEIGHT CHARTS FOR CHILDREN

Growth charts help you check whether your child is developing as expected. The solid green and purple percentile lines identify average height or weight at a given age, the dotted red and orange lines indicate the high and low ends of the normal range. Ninety-six percent of all children's height or weight falls within the dotted lines. To monitor your child's development, request a chart from your pediatrician.

GROWTH CURVES
Your child's measurements, when plotted regularly, should form a natural curve roughly parallel to the average (50th percentile). Children generally progress in line with their height and weight at birth. For example, if your child's height is above average at birth, then his or her weight curve will also fall above the central one. There should be cause for concern only if the growth pattern veers away from the average curve.

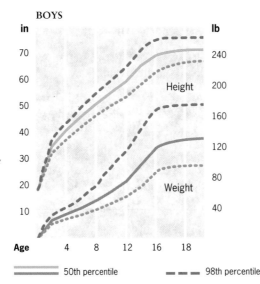

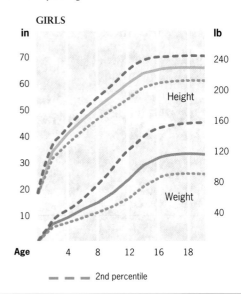

50th percentile ----- 98th percentile ----- 2nd percentile

128

Improving the Household's Diet with a

Family Conference

The best way to rethink the family diet is through teamwork. Get everyone in the household involved by calling a conference. Turn the meeting into a special occasion that will be fun and enjoyed by all.

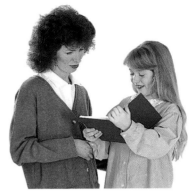

The place: the family kitchen or dining table. The time: a weekend hour or weekday evening when everyone can arrange to be free and at home. The refreshments: a medley of the family's favorite snacks.

The supplies: blank paper and felt-tip pens or pencils in different colors.

Appoint a note taker. Label different sheets of paper: Likes, Dislikes, Eat More, Eat Less, Special Needs, Healthy Snacks, and Special Treats.

VALUABLE COMMUNICATION
Making time for a family discussion is a good way of looking at the healthy—and unhealthy—aspects of everyone's diet.

HOLDING THE CONFERENCE

Start talking! Discuss the way the family usually eats. Give everyone a chance to list his or her favorite foods, dishes, and types of cooking, as well as the things he or she likes the least.

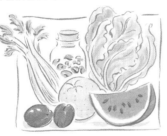

1 *Let everyone come up with suggestions for healthy foods that the family should eat more of, then a list of the items that should be cut down or eliminated altogether.*

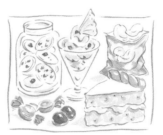

2 *Talk about the fun foods that everybody loves but are too high in fats, sugars, and certain additives to be truly healthy. Agree how often and when these special treats can be eaten.*

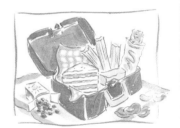

3 *Think about how to maintain the family's eating patterns away from home—the children's packed lunches or school meals, the adults' lunches at work or on business trips.*

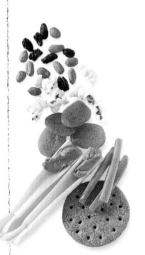

COMPETITION TIME
Ask for suggestions for healthy snacks to have on hand. Reward the family member who can contribute the greatest number of ideas.

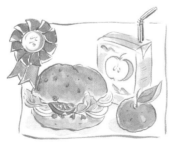

4 *Give a prize to the person who comes up with the best ideas for healthy eating in these situations— including suggestions by the family's junior members for foods to pack in their school lunch boxes that will not be traded or left uneaten.*

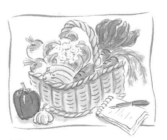

5 *Agree to try a new healthy recipe at regular intervals. Make up a menu-planning rotation so that each person helps the household cook to think up the menus for a week's meals, work out the shopping lists, and shop for the ingredients.*

BREAKFAST STRATEGY TIPS

▶ *Discuss the elements that make up a healthy breakfast; think about foods that are the easiest to put together when everyone is in a hurry.*

▶ *Simplify breakfast preparation in the morning by planning ahead—for example, set the table and put out dry cereals the night before.*

SPECIAL DIETS

A high proportion of the population follows some kind of special diet. Many people do so to lose weight, but a significant number follow a program for medical reasons.

Special diets tend to fall into one of three broad categories. The first is the exclusion diet—particular foods are not eaten because of a food allergy or intolerance—for example, the gluten-free diet prescribed for people with celiac disease or the diet that excludes cow's milk products for lactose-intolerant individuals. The second category is the reduced-intake diet, in which less is eaten of certain elements that are likely to aggravate an existing health problem, such as a low-salt diet for people who are prone to hypertension. The third regimen is an increased-consumption diet in which an individual eats more of foods that are believed to confer specific health benefits. For example, nutritional guidelines for postmenopausal women at risk of developing osteoporosis include an increased consumption of high-calcium foods, such as low-fat cheeses and milk, sardines and salmon (with the bones), dried peas, and leafy green vegetables.

GLUTEN-FREE DIET

One of the most common special diets is the gluten-free regimen, prescribed for people who suffer from an extreme sensitivity to various grains. Gluten—a protein found in wheat, barley, rye, and oats—is impossible for some people to absorb. A person's inability to absorb gluten, whether because of celiac disease or any one of a number of related medical conditions, causes thickening and inflammation of the small bowel, which prevents the absorption of nutrients. The problem is controlled by eliminating the offending grains from the diet.

People with this sensitivity must cut out a wide range of foodstuffs, including all standard varieties of bread and pasta and most breakfast cereals. They must also become scrupulous and knowledgeable readers of food package labels. Gluten in the form of "wheat," "flour," "wheat starch," "modified starch" and similar substances is a common additive in a variety of processed foods. It even turns up in canned soups and bottled sauces, although not every manufacturer uses it. Celiac sufferers rapidly learn which brands to avoid, and organizations set up to support and advise people with this condition frequently publish lists of gluten-free products as well as recipes for bread substitutes and other dishes.

But even people with a high sensitivity to wheat need complex carbohydrates in their diet. Digestible carbohydrates in a gluten-free diet may come from grains like rice or corn, which do not contain this particular protein. Health food stores and some supermarkets stock gluten-free breads, pastas, and crackers, such as ricecakes, that can take the place of the forbidden foods.

TREATING ARTHRITIS

Some naturopaths recommend a high-alkaline diet to reduce the toxic acids that they believe accumulate in the joints of people suffering from arthritis. This regimen, not among the arthritis treatments normally advocated by orthodox medicine, bans many of the same substances, such as wheat flour and its derivatives, forbidden to people on gluten-free diets. It may also eliminate or severely curtail the intake of cow's milk, citrus fruits, salt, pepper, and meat. In fact, becoming vegetarian has helped many arthritics.

Some sufferers have found that avoiding all foods of the nightshade family—tomatoes, potatoes, and eggplant—eases symptoms, though others have not succeeded with this approach.

Many people with arthritis have claimed that eating boiled stinging nettle leaves brings relief. A tea made with the leaves of the nettle or herbs of the mint family, such as basil, oregano, and rosemary, is also recommended.

EASING INFLAMMATION Pineapples contain an enzyme called bromelain, which is thought to reduce the inflammation caused by arthritis. Oily fish may also be helpful.

THE DIABETIC DIET

Diabetes is another medical condition that requires a controlled diet. There are different kinds of diabetes, but their common denominator is a disruption of the body's ability to metabolize carbohydrates because of difficulties in the production of insulin, a hormone that controls the amount of sugar in the blood (see page 48). A small percentage of diabetics need regular insulin injections, but most, especially those who have adult-onset diabetes, can stabilize their condition through diet.

Diabetics are often advised to schedule their intake of food in accordance with the times of maximum insulin activity within the body, eating small meals of carefully controlled quantities at regular intervals throughout the day. They must also restrict their intake of added sugar; a common guideline is to limit their consumption to less than 5 percent of their total daily caloric intake. To accommodate the needs of this relatively large segment of the population, food manufacturers now produce an extensive range of sugar-free products.

Obesity often goes hand in hand with diabetes, and for many diabetics a calorie-controlled weight-reduction diet and a regular exercise regimen are fundamental to managing their condition. In general, the dietary recommendations for diabetics conform closely to the nutritional guidelines put forward by the American Heart Association: a reduction of total fats in the diet to less than 30 percent of all calories consumed, with saturated fats reduced to less than 10 percent; a reduction in the intake of salt, high-cholesterol foods, and alcohol; and a substantial increase in unrefined complex carbohydrates, for example, those found in brown rice and whole-grain breads and crackers, to about 55 percent of total calories.

CUTTING DOWN ON SALT

Some special diets include a reduction in the intake of sodium, a component of salt and other ingredients.

Excessive salt in the diet is one of a number of factors believed to be associated with the development of hypertension. Obesity, high alcohol consumption, smoking, a stressful job or lifestyle, and heredity have also been implicated. Even though scientists have not yet been able to provide sufficient ironclad evidence that eating too much salt is a direct cause of hypertension, many studies have shown that a reduction in salt will help to decrease high blood pressure. Virtually everyone treated for hypertension is told to cut down on their intake of salt.

continued on page 133

Washing added salt away
The added salt content of processed foods can be significantly reduced by rinsing them in running water. A study at Duke University in North Carolina revealed that canned green beans rinsed for 1 minute, lost 41 percent of their sodium. The same treatment removed 76 percent of the salt added to canned tuna.

SODIUM CONTENT IN CONDIMENTS AND SEASONINGS

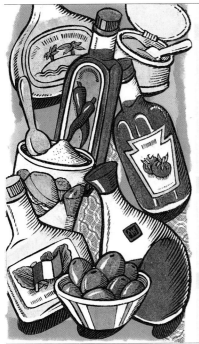

FOOD ITEM	AMOUNT	SODIUM (mg)
SEASONINGS		
Table salt	1 tsp	2,100
Baking powder	1 tsp	339
Chili powder	1 tsp	26
Garlic salt	1 tsp	2,050
Horseradish	1 tbs	165
Meat tenderizer	1 tsp	1,680
Mustard, prepared Dijon	1 tsp	126
Green olives	4	323
Onion salt	1 tsp	1,620
SAUCES		
Chili	1 tbsp	227
Ketchup	1 tbsp	168
Soy	1 tbsp	1,029
Tabasco	1 tspp	66
Worcestershire	1 tbsp	147
SALAD DRESSINGS		
French	1 tbsp	214
Mayonnaise	1 tbsp	78
Thousand Island	1 tbsp	109

The Heart Attack Survivor

Even a mild heart attack is a terrifying event for the patients and their families. It gives many survivors all the motivation they need to make fundamental and radical improvements in their diet and general lifestyle. Learning to eat healthfully is essential for preventing further damage to the heart and for enjoying an active life.

George is a 45-year-old optician who runs his own practice. His wife, Charlotte, works with him. One morning after a heavy snowfall, George began to shovel the snow off the pavement in front of his premises. But before he finished the task, he collapsed with severe chest pains and was taken to the hospital, where doctors diagnosed a heart attack. Fortunately, the attack was a relatively mild one, and George was told that after a period of rest and recovery, he should be able to resume work. However, his family doctor gave him a severe lecture about the need to change his eating habits, especially by cutting down on saturated fats. He put George on a low-fat diet and warned him of the grave risks he would take if he failed to stick to it.

WHAT SHOULD GEORGE DO?

George and Charlotte should eat plenty of fresh vegetables and complex carbohydrates. If they want to grill something quickly during the week, they could choose a lean fish such as flounder, which is free of saturated fats. Their customary Sunday lunch has usually featured roast beef with roast potatoes. Since George and Charlotte have more time and energy for cooking on Sundays, this day presents a good opportunity to experiment with vegetarian recipes to substitute for the usual roast. Sandwiches for their weekday lunches should have fillings low in saturated fat, such as sardines mixed with a dash of lemon juice or vinegar. George should also avoid eating heavy meals within two hours of going to bed.

DIET
Red meats, even after trimming, contain considerable saturated fat. Whole-milk dairy products can also be harmful.

COOKING METHODS
Certain cooking techniques increase fat consumption. Frying is the highest-fat method, closely followed by roasting if the meat is basted with drippings.

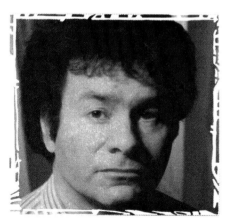

FITNESS
Self-employed people may have little leisure time for keeping fit and relaxing.

Action Plan

DIET
Cut back on beef (the white meat of turkey is a leaner substitute). Eat more oily fish, such as herring. Use low-fat dairy products, such as reduced-fat mozzarella cheese.

COOKING METHODS
Try some alternative cooking techniques such as poaching skinless chicken or turkey breast. Boil or bake potatoes. Microwave, poach, or steam fish rather than frying it.

FITNESS
Start exercising regularly, but gently. Possibilities to explore include walking, swimming, gardening, and yoga.

HOW THINGS TURN OUT FOR GEORGE

George has recently been back to the doctor for a checkup and seems to be making a good recovery. Although fish and fresh salads now play a substantial part on the weekly menu, Charlotte still feels that she and her husband are eating too much meat. She has tried replacing the Sunday roast with vegetarian alternatives but to no avail. She suspects this may be a losing battle. They have agreed, however, to one meatless meal per week.

The body needs only the amount of sodium found in about 1 gram of salt per day to function normally. Nutritional guidelines in many countries suggest that even people who are not at risk of hypertension should limit their daily consumption to a maximum of 3 grams (3,000 milligrams, or 1½ teaspoons). People with high blood pressure should cut their intake even further.

A hidden ingredient

Sticking to a low-salt diet requires diligent attention. Many people salt their food—some do this before they've tasted it—but salt also has a way of sneaking into our food. In the United States, for instance, researchers have established that salt added at the table accounts for only one-third of an individual's average consumption. The other two-thirds is eaten in processed foods. But salty snacks, such as potato chips or pretzels, are not the only culprits.

Salt has long been used as a preservative to keep food safe. Salted or smoked fish, pickled vegetables, and cured meats—such as bacon and salami—have always contained salt to keep them from spoiling. In fact, government food standards specify quantities of salt for many foods, such as sausages. Manufacturers rely heavily—most nutritionists would say too heavily—upon salt to enhance flavor. Canned vegetables and vegetable juices, both canned and dried soups and sauces, canned beans and fish, and many breakfast cereals include salt and other forms of sodium; so, too, do milk and cheeses. You should always read the label before you buy. Many manufacturers now supply low-salt or no-added-salt versions of their products.

In any purchase of packaged food, the low-salt shopper needs to read carefully the small print on the label. As well as noting the quantity of salt itself, watch out for sodium hiding in other ingredients: MSG (monosodium glutamate), soy sauce, baking powder, hydrolyzed vegetable protein, miso, bouillon, kelp and other seaweed products, sodium citrate, and such additives as the sweetener saccharin.

Learning to like less salt

The best strategy for cutting down on salt is to reeducate your taste buds to enjoy other natural flavors in food. By gradually reducing the amount of salt you add to food over a

---

SEASONING WITHOUT SALT

In the kitchen, make use of ingredients that provide flavor but no sodium. Draw upon garlic, onions, gingerroot, vinegar, wine, fiery chili peppers, and the juice of lemons, oranges, and other fruits. If you must use a prepared condiment, stick to lower-salt varieties or improvise salt-reduced substitutions: Worcestershire sauce, for instance, though hardly salt free, has much less sodium than most soy sauces and packs an equally aromatic punch.

ENHANCING FLAVOR
By choosing highly aromatic herbs and spices, you can add interest to meat dishes without noticing the loss of salt.

Dill

Bay leaves

Rosemary

Cumin seeds

Thyme

Mint

Star anise

Red wine, vinegar, and lemon juice

Garlic cloves

Red and green chilies

Sage

Curry powder

Gingerroot

Onion

Tarragon

---

period of days or weeks, you will become more sensitive to saltiness. After a few weeks of progressively decreasing the use of the salt shaker, an amount that would have once seemed just normal will make the food taste unpleasantly salty. Experiment with flavorful seasonings (see box above).

On a low-salt diet you face a challenge when eating in restaurants. Choose dishes that can be cooked to order, and ask the kitchen to prepare it without adding salt.

LOWERING CHOLESTEROL

If you are following a low-cholesterol diet, you have to be equally resolute. To cut down on the saturated fats that are the building blocks of the health-threatening type of cholesterol, you will have to banish certain foods from everyday use. Such dairy products as whole milk and butter are perilously high in saturated fats; they should be replaced by their low-fat or fat-free counterparts, for example, skim milk. You can replace butter with polyunsaturated vegetable oils or olive oil, which is substantially monounsaturated (see page 51).

Holding the salt

Cut down on the quantities of salt called for in recipes. In a recipe designed to serve four people, ¼ teaspoon of salt will add 0.13 grams (133 milligrams) of sodium to each helping. A tablespoon of salt in a dish of the same size will add 1.6 gram (1,600 milligrams) to every diner's salt intake—over a quarter of the maximum recommended quota for the day.

USING FOOD
TO LOSE WEIGHT

A weight-loss diet, in essence, is simply one in which the body takes in less energy in the form of calories than it expends. But there is nothing simple about the diet industry.

Hundreds upon thousands of magazine and newspaper articles, as well as a vast array of diet books, hold out the promise of delivering surefire methods for shedding fat and decreasing weight. Every city or town has its diet clubs and franchised vendors of "foolproof" weight-reduction schemes. Manufacturers of special diet foods—from liquid high-protein meal substitutes to appetite-killing confectionery bars and snacks—make extravagant claims in order to sell hope to weight-conscious consumers. A few of these diets are based on sound nutritional advice. But many companies make exaggerated or overly optimistic claims.

People who follow recommendations to cut down on calories will lose weight, but it is easy to put the weight back on again if, out of boredom or hunger or for some other reason, you give up the diet.

THE LOW-CALORIE DIET

For generations of dieters, one of the most familiar regimens has been the low-calorie diet, which concentrates simply on cutting down the number of calories consumed on a day-to-day basis. Its adherents rarely let a mouthful pass their lips without first consulting a chart detailing the exact caloric intake for every single ingredient.

Calorie control is, indeed, important for anyone trying to lose weight, but the major failing of such a diet is its lack of emphasis on the need for a varied and balanced intake of foods to provide the full range of health-sustaining nutrients your body requires.

Low-calorie diets offer little to deter a rigid calorie counter with a sweet tooth, for instance, from abandoning a dinner in favor of a large slab of thickly frosted chocolate cake. This is justified on the premise that the individual has not exceeded the recommended maximum calories for the day. Nutritionists would not be surprised to discover that this extreme interpretation of calorie control failed to deliver the dieter's hoped-for weight loss or to find the dieter complaining of low energy, irritability, constipation, or vertigo.

FAT DISTRIBUTION IN MEN AND WOMEN

About 10 to 15 percent of a man's weight consists of fat, while 20 to 25 percent is average for most women. Fat is stored under the skin all over the body but it is most likely to accumulate on specific areas of the male and female bodies.

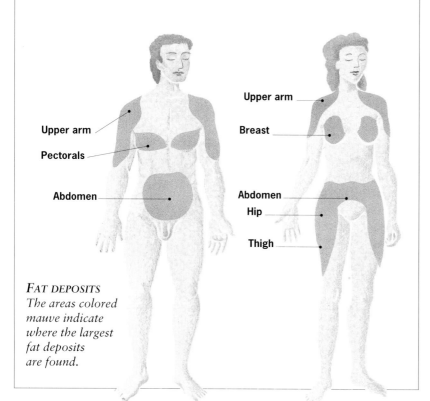

Upper arm

Pectorals

Abdomen

Upper arm

Breast

Abdomen

Hip

Thigh

FAT DEPOSITS
The areas colored mauve indicate where the largest fat deposits are found.

BREAKING DOWN FAT

The places that fat settles in our bodies and the speed at which the body burns it up are controlled by hormones. Estrogen, the female sex hormone, mainly governs the deposits of fat around the hips and thighs, while insulin—generated in the body via the consumption of carbohydrates—dictates the deposit of fat around the neck, shoulder blades, and abdomen.

The body is an efficient ecosystem, however, and is constantly recycling its fat stores to provide the energy it needs. Two stress hormones, adrenaline and noradrenaline, are responsible for releasing stored fat reserves when fresh energy is required.

When these stress hormones go into operation, the fat deposits in certain parts of the body, such as the abdomen or the face, which are more sensitive to their presence, are recycled more readily and are the first to begin disappearing. For this reason, when weight loss does occur, the first visible signs for both males and females are likely to be a thinner face and a flatter stomach.

THE SPOT-REDUCTION DIET

A weight-loss program that from time to time has been fashionable is the so-called spot-reduction diet. It promises the removal of unwanted excess fat from particular "problem" areas, such as the buttocks or hips, through a combination of low-fat diet and an exercise program.

People who cut their consumption of fat and increase the amount of exercise they do will indeed have a good chance of losing weight since fats—gram for gram—deliver a far heavier cargo of calories than the same quantity of protein or carbohydrate. But the notion that such a dieter can sculpt his or her body by a highly localized weight-reduction program is wishful thinking.

Scientists at King's College, London, set up a study to compare the effectiveness of a spot-reduction diet to that of a standard weight-reduction diet that allowed a controlled daily intake of 1,000 to 1,200 calories. They asked two groups of women to follow each regimen and then compared the results. Both groups lost poundage, but the weight loss followed the same pattern: most inches were lost from the waist rather than from the hips or thighs, as promised in the spot-reduction plan, and the women's busts became smaller as quickly as their hips did.

FOOD-COMBINING DIET

Another eating plan that is enjoying a surge of popularity is food-combining. This system operates by a strict set of rules governing the types of food that may—or may not—be eaten within the same meal. Weight loss is only a single aspect of the diet, which also claims to promote general good health.

By eating or avoiding certain foods at certain times, the dieter supposedly purges the body of harmful toxins and restores the fragile balance of acidity and alkalinity in the body's internal chemistry.

The central tenet of food-combining is that protein foods, such as meat or beans, and starchy ones, such as potatoes or rice, are incompatible: eating them in a single meal is thought to wreak havoc with the digestive system and prevent the proper absorption of nutrients. Therefore a stew that incorporates meat and potatoes, a breakfast of cereal and milk, or a sandwich pairing bread with cheese, meat, eggs, or fish would be out of bounds. The combinations of grains and legumes, which are crucial sources of essential protein for vegans and vegetarians, would also be discouraged.

Other rules include banning fruit from meals and eating it only on its own as a separate meal or snack, and rejecting all processed foods. Taken literally, this rule would mean that even 100 percent whole-grain bread baked from organic flours could not be included in the diet.

Scientists dismiss this system as a fad based on nutritional and physiological misconceptions. Most basic foods contain a combination of starches and proteins. The digestive tract does not distinguish between them, and the body is perfectly competent to process them when they arrive in the stomach at the same time.

The body also has its own internal mechanism for balancing acidity and alkalinity and for ridding itself of most naturally occurring toxins.

continued on page 138

The changing shape of women

Perceptions of the "ideal" female shape have changed many times throughout the course of history.

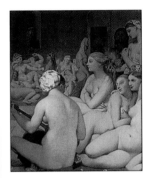

THE ROUNDED FIGURE *During the 18th century, an ample, curvy figure was often perceived by artists as representing female beauty.*

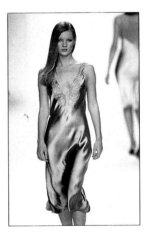

THE SLIM FIGURE *In the 20th century, perceptions of the ideal woman's body ranged from the well-endowed Marilyn Monroe to the slender figure of the model Kate Moss.*

The Dietitian

A dietitian's unique skill is to translate the science of nutrition into practical information about food. Dietitians advise people on dietary treatments for specific conditions, such as obesity or kidney disease, and about eating healthfully.

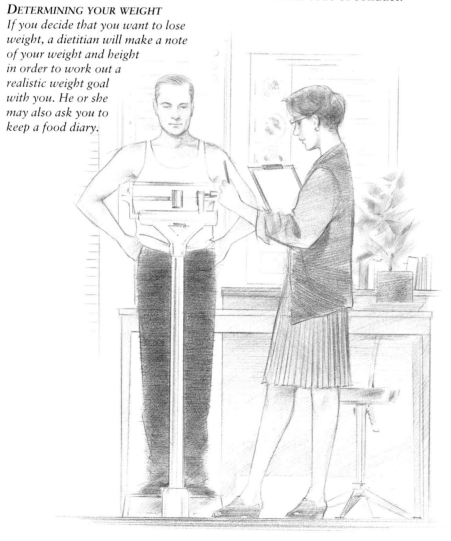

A QUESTION OF BALANCE
A dietitian will help you to achieve and maintain good health through a balanced diet that is personally tailored to meet your needs.

DETERMINING YOUR WEIGHT
If you decide that you want to lose weight, a dietitian will make a note of your weight and height in order to work out a realistic weight goal with you. He or she may also ask you to keep a food diary.

Degree-qualified and registered dietitians advise clients on their dietary needs. They often provide consultations at their own clinics, but they may also work as part of a team, caring for people in a hospital or in the community. They work to a strict ethical code of conduct.

What is the difference between a nutritionist and a dietitian?
Although many nutritionists are qualified in nutrition, not all practitioners have taken courses that are recognized by academic or government bodies. Dietitians, on the other hand, have an advanced degree in nutrition and have studied physiology and biochemistry in preparation for state registration in dietetics. Their courses include practical training in hospital and community settings, approved by the Dietitians' Board of the Council for Professions Supplementary to Medicine (CPSM).

Do I need a referral from my doctor to see a dietitian?
If you want general dietary assessment, weight control advice, healthy eating information, or guidance on sports nutrition, no referral is necessary. But there are some disorders that require dietary treatment as part of their overall management, and for these you need a referral from a doctor or dentist. These conditions include obesity and eating disorders; heart disease; food allergies; raised cholesterol; kidney and liver disease; celiac disease; gastrointestinal disorders, such as irritable bowel syndrome, ulcerative colitis, and constipation; diabetes; and some types of cancer.

If I decide to lose weight, what will a dietitian ask me?
A dietitian will ask you about your current eating habits and lifestyle—for example, how often you eat, your

food likes and dislikes, and whether you have any special dietary needs. You may be asked about your previous dieting experiences.

What do dietitians recommend as a healthful way to lose weight?

A dietitian will suggest that you follow a balanced diet with a variety of healthful foods. A recommended diet would aim at reducing your normal daily caloric intake by about 500 calories. For example, if you eat 2,000 calories, you should reduce your intake to 1,500 calories. (Women should not go below about 1,200 calories a day, and men should not go below about 1,500 calories.)

Rather than having you count calories, the dietitian will help you to plan ways to lower your fat intake, particularly fried foods and fatty foods such as pastry, mayonnaise, and cookies. Keeping a food diary will help you to be more aware of your eating habits and give you a basis for making gradual changes. In addition, you will be encouraged to include regular exercise (for example, three to four times a week for 20 to 40 minutes or walking for 2 or more miles) to help maintain your metabolic rate and preserve or increase your lean tissue (muscle). All together, the amount of weight you should lose is no more than ½ to 2 pounds per week; otherwise, you will become too hungry and start losing lean tissue.

Will I need to take vitamin and mineral supplements?

A well-balanced diet should provide you with all the vitamins and minerals you need. It should be based on fresh fruits, vegetables, whole-grain cereals, low-fat protein foods, including dairy products. Because it may be difficult to obtain enough iron, calcium, magnesium, zinc, riboflavin, B_6, and folic acid if your intake dips below 1,200 to 1,500 calories a day, the dietitian may advise, as a precaution, a multivitamin and mineral supplement to help ensure that you are meeting your nutrient requirements in full. But aim first to get as many vitamins and minerals as you can from your food.

How often will I need to visit the dietitian to check my weight-loss progress?

Time between visits will vary from one to four weeks. Frequent appointments will help to keep you motivated. If you cannot make regular appointments, ask your spouse or a friend to help check your weight and give you some encouragement. But your dietitian will be able to give you more detailed advice each time you go, talk over any specific dietary problems you have, and discuss ways to help you to continue to improve your eating habits.

After I have reached the right weight, how long do I have to continue the weight-loss diet?

Once you have reached your healthy weight, you will be advised to gradually increase your calorie intake over

a period of one to two weeks by eating larger quantities of low-fat, high-carbohydrate foods, for example, pasta. If you have made gradual and practical changes, you will find it easy not to go back to your old eating habits. Continue to eat the same well-balanced meals that you did when you were dieting, and check your weight about every two weeks.

WHAT YOU CAN DO AT HOME

Most people who genuinely want to control their weight will take enough positive steps toward improvement. But there is little merit in trying to change old eating patterns overnight, sweeping everything from butter to pizza to chocolate cookies out of your life and kitchen forever in a single, irrevocable act. The most effective changes are the ones that you make gradually—they may soon become just a habit.

1 *Eat less butter, margarine, and mayonnaise on sandwiches. Eat fewer fried foods like french fries and doughnuts; fatty meats and meat products such as steaks, sausages, and hamburgers; pastry dishes and pies; cakes, cookies, and puddings; chocolate; potato chips and other snacks.*

2 *Change to lower-fat alternatives: skim or low-fat milk instead of whole milk; poultry without skin and the white meat rather than the dark; fish instead of red meat; trimmed lean meat instead of marbled; low-fat cheese instead of Cheddar or a hard cheese such as Parmesan; broiled, steamed, stir-fried, or baked food instead of fried.*

MAKING A CHICKEN LEG LESS FATTY
Chicken skin contains a lot of saturated fat, so remove it before cooking. Using a pair of scissors, snip the edge of the chicken skin, then pull the chicken skin away from the meat.

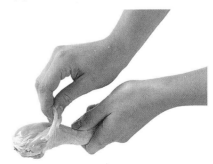

Can food burn fat?
Some diets tout the weight-reducing powers of particular foods. Nutritionists tend to dismiss these as fad or folklore.

Grapefruit, for instance, has been promoted as a dieter's best friend, on the grounds that the acid or the enzymes in this fruit actually burn up body fat. With its high vitamin C content, grapefruit, like all fruit, is a valuable addition to any diet. But the notion that it can cut through fat in the same way that detergents cut through grease is erroneous.

HIDDEN FATS IN YOUR FOOD

Cutting down on excess fat and calories becomes much easier once you know where the fats are lurking. It is important, therefore, to analyze the components of individual dishes to see how much fat they really contain.

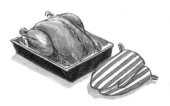

ROAST CHICKEN
Sixty-two percent of the calories in a serving of roast chicken comes from the fat in the skin.

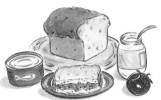

TUNA SANDWICH
Just over half the calories in a tuna, tomato, and mayonnaise sandwich comes from the fat in the mayonnaise.

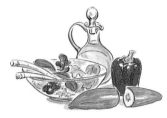

DRESSED SALAD
Ninety percent of the calories in a green salad tossed with an oily or creamy dressing comes from the fat in the dressing rather than from the salad greens.

Not all popular diet systems deserve outright rejection. Any plan that features a healthy balance of different foods, emphasizes the consumption of fresh fruits, vegetables, and grains, and encourages a reduced intake of calories and saturated fats is sending a helpful message for healthy eating.

HARMING THE BODY
Certain diets, however, not only are lacking in benefits to health but also may actively endanger it. For instance, liquid diet formulas, if they are substituted for all or most regular meals, deliver speedy weight loss but ultimately are harmful to the body. They tend to be extremely low in calories—some provide no more than 300 to 500 calories per day—but excessively high in protein. A person sticking to such a diet will lose weight but will simultaneously upset the balance of her endocrine system. Production of some essential hormones will be diminished, and this decrease may cause a variety of unpleasant symptoms, ranging from constipation and abdominal bloating to nausea, dizziness, and fatigue. Studies reveal that people who try these diets do lose weight but almost inevitably regain it.

For some dieters the health risk is even greater. A sudden switch away from this type of regimen and back to a normal diet could result in a rapid drop in the levels of potassium and magnesium in the blood. These minerals help maintain the heart's normal rhythm, and in rare cases such a disturbance could be fatal.

Fasting—literally starving to lose weight—is a dangerous practice. If the body is not supplied with nutrients, it will exhaust its stores of fat then begin to digest its own muscles—including cardiac muscle, which can lead to heart failure. Other risks include gout and vitamin-deficiency illnesses.

All crash diets have their perils. Bones can be weakened through lack of minerals, and nutritional imbalances may lead to the development of gallstones or even heart disease. Finally, these efforts interfere with the body's own normal weight-control mechanisms, with the result that any weight lost in this manner is likely to be gained back faster and more easily than it would have been if no crash diet had ever been attempted.

The only safe, healthy, and reliable way to lose weight is to do it slowly and gradually, with a permanent adjustment of eating habits, accompanied by an increase in energy expenditure through regular exercise.

The fashionable body
Many people who attempt a weight-reduction diet do not, in fact, need to lose weight. Women especially suffer from the modern Western culture's obsession with a slim, boyish, willowy figure. They often believe themselves to be overweight when by any medical standard they are not. Skeletal fashion models parade down the runways. Film

actresses who are anything other than lean are virtually never seen as romantic heroines. The clothes on sale in many trendy shops are available only in sizes that exclude virtually half the female population, as are those portrayed in fashion magazines.

For some emotionally vulnerable people, especially adolescent girls, this cult of fanatical slenderness combines with psychological problems such as low self-esteem to precipitate potentially life-threatening eating disorders like anorexia nervosa. Anorexics believe themselves to be fat, even when visibly emaciated, and starve themselves to get even thinner. Long-term effects include a damaged immune system, anemia, heart disease and osteoporosis. Another eating disorder, bulimia, is characterized by a pattern of bingeing on food, followed by self-induced vomiting or massive doses of laxatives. Repeated vomiting may inflame the esophagus and dehydrate the body.

There are, indeed, many adults—and children—in the affluent Western world who are to some degree overweight, even obese. And because of sedentary lifestyles and unhealthy diets, the number continues to rise. The National Health and Nutritional Examination Survey (NHANES) III data show a 34 percent incidence of obesity, up from 29 percent. The incidence is higher in women than in men.

A moderate amount of excess poundage is not the same as obesity, and it is important to distinguish between the two.

CHANGING HABITS

A substantial number of calories can be eliminated by reviewing everyday eating habits. Change to low-fat milk, preferably skim. Use salad dressings sparingly, or make your own with less oil. Replace fried potatoes with baked or boiled, and eat potato chips only as a special treat, if ever. Increase the number of servings of vegetables and fruits and avoid cream sauces on them. Reduce the size of servings of meat and poultry and replace them with eggs, fish, or cooked dried beans for a few meals each week. Serve salad as a main dish and, when possible, use low-fat cheeses. Cut out high-fat drinks, desserts, and snacks, and watch what you put on your bread.

Dried fruits have a role in healthy eating, although they are high in sugar and so cannot be eaten with quite the same freedom as the fresh varieties. An unsweetened breakfast cereal, for instance, is tastier with a sprinkling of raisins or other chopped dried fruit. The fruit supplies not only sweetness but fiber, vitamins, and minerals. Since even a 1-ounce serving of conventionally sweetened commercial breakfast cereal may contain as many as 4 teaspoons of sugar, it is highly preferable to "sweeten" a serving of unsweetened breakfast cereal with the extra nutrition that even a few raisins can add.

For many people the idea of eliminating certain treat foods—ice cream, for example, or chocolate—drives them to guilty binges on these very foods. But by allowing one modest and carefully rationed indulgence every day—a single sweet cookie, a small slice of cake, or a few spoonfuls of ice cream—it is possible to forestall any desperate cravings. Give yourself an allowance of pleasurable foods every day, but limit this to one treat only—a croissant for breakfast, a cookie after lunch, or icecream at dinner—but not all three.

continued on page 142

DO YOU NEED TO LOSE WEIGHT?

In a society obsessed with slim figures, an individual may feel pressured to lose weight even when he is well within the range considered healthy for his age and height

One simple indicator of excess body fat is the waist to hip ratio, which can show the presence of fat on the abdomen. For women a ratio higher than 0.8 indicates that there is excessive abdominal fat. For men the crucial maximum is 0.95. If your ratio is higher than this, you may be well advised to lose some weight.

1 *To determine your waist-hip ratio, use a tape measure to find out the circumference of your waist, including any protruding stomach.*

2 *Repeat the above process to measure the circumference of your hips.*

3 *Divide the measurement of the waist by the hip measurement. The result is your waist-hip ratio.*

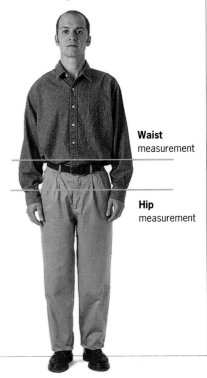

Waist measurement

Hip measurement

Cooking for a
Low-Fat Diet

For those who genuinely want to control their weight or improve their general health, the surest path to success lies in the ability to make basic, permanent changes in eating habits and attitudes.

ESSENTIAL UTENSILS
Nonstick pots and pans radically reduce the amount of cooking oil needed for sautéing meats and vegetables, cooking pancakes and omelets, and reheating cooked food.

Successful dieting requires a combination of nutritional knowledge and self-discipline. You need to know which foods are fattening and have a sound sense of caloric content as well as portion size control.

To remain healthy and well nourished, you should eat a wide variety of fresh foods in well-balanced combinations. This type of eating pattern will help you to avoid an excess of those elements, like saturated fats, that are detrimental both to your health and to the success of your diet.

It also helps, strange as it may seem, to enjoy good food, to plan meals creatively, and to look forward to them as a source not just of nourishment but also of positive pleasure.

MAKING THE RIGHT CUTS

Before cooking fatty cuts of meat, such as a lamb or pork chop, remove the external fat.

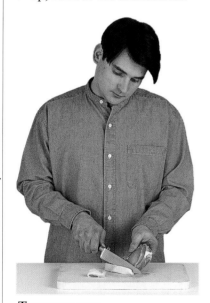

TRIMMING FAT
Using a sharp knife, trim off excess fat from around the chop. Do not remove all the fat, however, or the chop will lose its shape and moisture when cooked.

LIGHTLY DOES IT

A considerable saving of fat calories can be made by just a slight adjustment to preparation and cooking techniques. Even when you are using ordinary cookware, you can cut down on your use of oil.

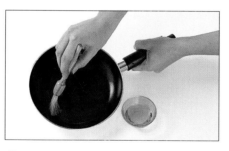

OILING WITH A BRUSH
Instead of pouring oil from the bottle straight into the frying pan, use an oil-dipped pastry brush or paper towel to apply a much lighter coating.

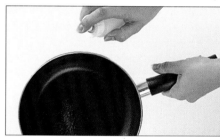

OILING WITH SPRAY
For a very fine coating of oil, use a non-aerosol oil spray. Hold the spray 6 inches away from the pan and give two to three squirts. Do not spray near flame.

CHOOSING LEAN MEAT

If you want the leanest beef, buy "choice" or "select" grades rather than "prime," which is the most marbled with fat.

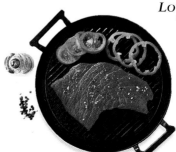

LOW-FAT CUTS
Trimmed loin and tenderloin of pork are leaner than ham. The flank and any part of the round are the leanest cuts of beef.

CUTTING BACK ON OIL

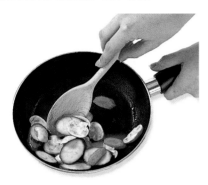

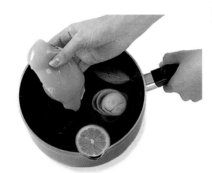

Spoon off and discard excess fat.

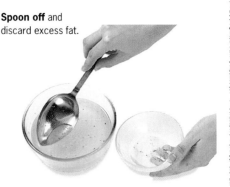

JUICE OR STOCK ALTERNATIVES
You can sauté some foods successfully by replacing the oil with a nonfat cooking liquid. Try simmering vegetables in tomato juice or fresh chicken stock that has been skimmed of all fat.

POACHING
Cook chicken or fish in a court bouillon —water acidulated with a little lemon juice or vinegar and seasoned with such herbs as fresh parsley, chervil, and thyme.

SKIMMING FAT
Prepare stocks, stews, roasts, and soups in advance and chill them for several hours or overnight. The fat within them will rise to the top and solidify and will be easy to remove. If you are in a hurry, float ice cubes, which will cause fat to solidify.

STEAMING VEGETABLES

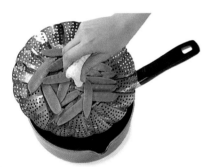

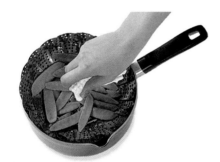

1 *A basket steamer that fits into a conventional saucepan is ideal for individual portions of vegetables. Keep the vegetables well-spaced in a single layer for even steaming.*

2 *Make sure the water in the saucepan is boiling before placing the basket steamer inside. There should be about 1 in of water to allow steaming, but it should not touch the vegetables.*

BAKING FISH

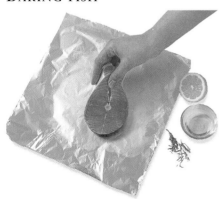

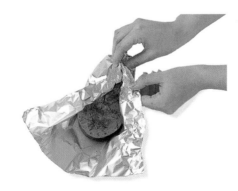

1 *A good alternative to frying fish is to bake it in aluminum foil. Lightly oil a square of foil and place the fish in the center. Sprinkle with lemon juice and fresh herbs such as dill.*

2 *Pull the edges of the foil up to cover the fish. Pinch the foil together to seal, then bake. Alternatively, bake the fish in parchment paper. Proceed as for foil but fold over the edges.*

QUICK TIPS FOR LESS FAT AND CHOLESTEROL

Here are a few ideas to help you reduce the amount of cholesterol in your diet.

▶ *Top a baked potato with low-fat cottage cheese and chives.*

▶ *Instead of sautéing mushrooms in butter, use a little Worcestershire sauce.*

▶ *Experiment with interesting whole-grain breads; many today also include seeds. They are usually so rich in flavor that they do not need to be spread with butter or margarine or mayonnaise.*

▶ *Instead of covering baked vegetable dishes with grated cheese, top with fresh whole-grain bread crumbs seasoned with herbs and drizzle a thimbleful of olive oil over the crumbs. Brown for a few minutes in the broiler to form a light, crispy topping.*

▶ *Puree cooked legumes to make a thick-textured soup instead of using cream or a roux sauce.*

▶ *Thicken sauces with vegetable purees, or use the purée as a sauce.*

▶ *When preparing hamburgers, make them with half ground beef and half ground turkey.*

Fast-food choices

A hamburger or fried-chicken restaurant does not have to be a dietary disaster area. Some chains, aware of the commercial advantage to be gained by catering to the growing number of weight-conscious consumers, now provide salad selections or special "healthy option" sections on their menus.

Even when choice is limited, it is possible to avoid excessive fat intake by choosing broiled chicken on a bun instead of deep-fried batter-coated chicken nuggets, or opting for a plain hamburger dressed with a little mustard or ketchup instead of one topped with melted cheese.

EATING OUT AND WATCHING YOUR WEIGHT

If all eating were done at home, weight control would be far more straightforward. But many people find the hardest part of maintaining a reasonable diet is eating in restaurants. When dining out, the restaurant you choose may make a vital difference in your ability to maintain your diet. A restaurant with an all-you-can-eat set-price buffet may be a good buy, but avoid it unless you are sure that some of the items on the heavily laden board are genuinely low-fat options.

Steakhouses famous for their giant cuts of marbled prime beef are generally unsuitable for anyone who wants to lose weight, as are old-fashioned restaurants specializing in the traditional butter-and-cream-based grande cuisine. In a large town or city, with many different cuisines available, the best course of action may be to choose a restaurant that serves food from a region or country known for its healthy diet.

In a Chinese or Japanese restaurant, for instance, a diligent dieter will find a wide selection of healthy, low-fat dishes: lightly cooked fresh fish; steamed rice topped with stir-fried vegetables and lean, slivered poultry; and light and crunchy salads. Italian restaurants can be another good choice, as long as heavily creamed pasta sauces are avoided in favor of tomato-based varieties, or if the pasta is tossed in a little olive oil and garlic and herbs (and if you use the Parmesan cheese sparingly). Restaurants that specialize in seafood are another good source of healthful options, but choose dishes that are broiled or steamed, not fried.

Any type of establishment worth a visit should be able to accommodate the needs of weight-conscious customers. If booking in advance, ask whether the menu includes any low-fat dishes or if the chef is willing, with a bit of notice, to prepare a dish with just a minimum of fat. In restaurants where all the food is cooked to order, there should be no difficulty in meeting special requests, such as having an accompanying sauce served on the side so that you can control the quantity that you use.

Many misguided diners imagine that they can save calories in advance by skipping lunch or starving themselves on the day of a restaurant dinner. In fact, the hungrier you are, the more likely you are to order—and consume—too much food or succumb to the richest temptations on the menu. One useful tactic is to eat a piece of fruit or some other low-fat snack just before leaving home. Then when you arrive at the restaurant, you will not feel ravenous; instead you will be ready to enjoy your meal.

EATING OUT: DIETER'S SURVIVAL TIPS

You do not have to give up all your social activities when trying to control your weight. Use the following tips to guide you through the high-calorie maze of dining out in restaurants.

▶ *Avoid fixed-price multicourse dinners. What you save in money you may pay for in excess calories. Choose from the à la carte menu, even if the individual dishes cost a little more, and limit yourself to the amount of food that you really need.*

▶ *Bear in mind that you do not have to eat all the food on your plate. If the portion is large, you can ask the waiter to have your meal divided in two and have one half wrapped for you to take home. Most restaurants are happy to cooperate.*

▶ *Do not choose your dessert until you have finished eating your main course: You will make a far more sensible choice than you might on an empty stomach.*

A LITTLE ON THE SIDE
Order your salad either with the dressing on the side or with cruets of vinegar and olive oil. Then you can dress the salad sparingly or with only a touch of oil. Most kitchens are overly generous with high-fat dressings.

CHAPTER 9

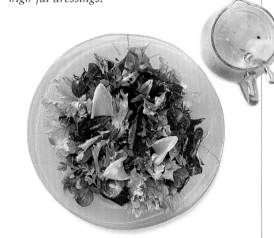

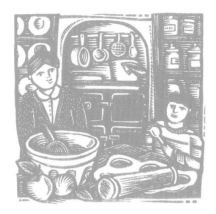

A HEALTHY KITCHEN

Food can be one of the great pleasures in life. Of course it should be properly selected, prepared, cooked, and stored to obtain optimum health benefits as well as enjoyment. Otherwise, vital nutrients may be lost or food wasted through spoilage. Safe and healthy cooking techniques are also important for safeguarding your family from food poisoning.

THE RAW MATERIALS

To get the most from your foods, learn all you can about how to buy, store, and handle them, so that they maintain their best qualities and are completely safe from contamination.

CHILLED FOODS

Developing good habits for safely refrigerating food is easy. Follow the tips below to help prevent food poisoning.

▶ *Refrigerate food as soon as possible. Cover or wrap all food, and never use unwashed containers. Also avoid reusing old plastic wrap, plastic bags, paper wrappings, or foil with fresh or frozen food.*

▶ *When thawing frozen foods, make sure that liquid does not drip on other food. The blood of raw meat and poultry should never be allowed to drip onto other foods because it is a major cause of food poisoning. Wrap meat carefully and place it on the lower shelves.*

▶ *Check the "use by" date. If the food is not dated and you cannot remember when it was refrigerated, throw it out.*

Cleanliness and proper food handling are of primary concern in the kitchen, because bacteria can multiply in its warm atmosphere at a prodigious rate, bringing with them the peril of food poisoning. The goal of kitchen hygiene is to reduce this risk to zero by giving bacteria as little opportunity for growth as possible.

If you have to delay serving food for an hour or two after it's been prepared, always store cold food in the refrigerator and keep hot food above 140°F. The hot food should have been thoroughly cooked to ensure that harmful bacteria were killed. This applies particularly to whole poultry and meats like rolled roasts, because bacteria can lurk in the center of these foods. Use a meat ther-mometer to check the food's temperature (see page 153). Ground meat, especially packaged hamburger, should also be cooked thoroughly (the center should be brown), because it can become contaminated with bacteria during the grinding process.

ROOM TEMPERATURE

Bacteria grow rapidly and produce toxins at temperatures between 60°F and 140°F. Therefore, cooked foods should never be left at room temperature for more than two hours. The warmer the temperature of the room, the shorter the time that food should be left standing. If the room's temperature is 90°F or higher, do not leave the food out for more than an hour, preferably not at all.

CLEANLINESS IN THE KITCHEN

Scrupulous hygiene is the key to a safe kitchen, but this is not as daunting as it sounds. The aim is not sterile operating-room standards but basic domestic hygiene. To achieve this, follow the steps outlined below.

▶ *Wash your hands with warm water and soap before preparing food, and clean all work surfaces daily using a disinfectant designed for food preparation areas.*

▶ *Wipe surfaces dry, as moisture provides a potential breeding ground for bacteria.*

▶ *Do not place cooked or ready-to-eat food on a surface that has had raw food on it unless you clean it thoroughly first. Raw food, particularly poultry, meat, and fish, is more likely to have bacteria on it, which will transfer to the cooked food.*

▶ *Wipe up food spills as they occur, using a clean cloth or paper towel. Use paper towels to mop up spills on the kitchen floor.*

▶ *Leave dishcloths to soak after use in a mild bleach solution, and change them every day to prevent bacteria from building up and contaminating surfaces with which the cloths come into contact.*

▶ *Whether you use an acrylic chopping board or a wooden one, you should pour boiling water over the board to sterilize it or soak it in a mild bleach solution for a minute. Rinse with clean water.*

CHOPPING SAFELY
Clean your knife and board thoroughly after chopping meat and before chopping vegetables.

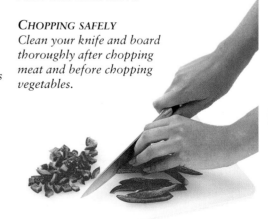

Animal products are especially susceptible to spoilage. Throw away any dairy, egg, meat, poultry, or fish dishes that have been at room temperature for more than two hours. Salads and pickled foods are less likely to spoil because their acid medium—vinegar or lemon juice—retards the development of bacteria. After storing leftover food in the refrigerator or freezer, reheat it to at least 165°F and serve while it is still hot.

REFRIGERATION

All perishable foods should be stored in the refrigerator. These include meat, fish, poultry, and dairy products, as well as berries and most vegetables. Keep raw meat, bacon, poultry, and fish in the coldest part of the refrigerator—usually the bottom shelf, though some appliances have a specially designated bin with a temperature regulator for these foods. Put cooked dishes on center shelves, and vegetables and salad greens in the bottom bins.

Carrots, turnips and most other root vegetables can be stored in the refrigerator. Potatoes and yams should be kept in a cool, dark cupboard, otherwise their starch turns to sugar. Tomatoes taste better if kept at room temperature, but must be used more quickly. Relishes, ketchup, salad dressing, and similar foods should go into the refrigerator once they have been opened, but are not overly perishable at room temperature.

Avoid overfilling a refrigerator because this blocks air circulation. For maximum efficiency, keep the temperature between 32°F and 41°F; if you doubt the accuracy, use a refrigerator thermometer in the coldest section to check on it. Before cleaning the refrigerator, remove all the foods and store the most perishable ones in an ice chest. Clean the refrigerator with a recommended cleaner or wipe surfaces with a solution of baking soda and warm water. Some household soaps and detergents may leave a smell behind that will taint the food.

FREEZER SAFETY

The low temperature of the freezer preserves the food and prevents nutritional loss by arresting bacterial activity that starts the decay. Freezers should be set at 0°F or below for rapid freezing and proper storage.

Wrap foods for freezing in freezer wrap or heavy-duty plastic bags or with aluminium foil. If using plastic containers, choose types that are about 3 inches tall or less. Leave some space at the top, and make sure they are securely covered. If foods are refrigerated or frozen in large, deep containers, the food in the middle stays warm longer, and bacteria can grow in this area.

Label packages with the contents and date. Most foods can be frozen safely providing they are well wrapped. But a few foods should not be frozen: eggs in their shells will crack, and milk will separate.

CONTROLLING HOUSEHOLD PESTS

The kitchen is a breeding ground for pests, which enter uninvited and damage cupboard contents, infect food, and spread disease. All pests need to be evicted. This chart shows what to do.

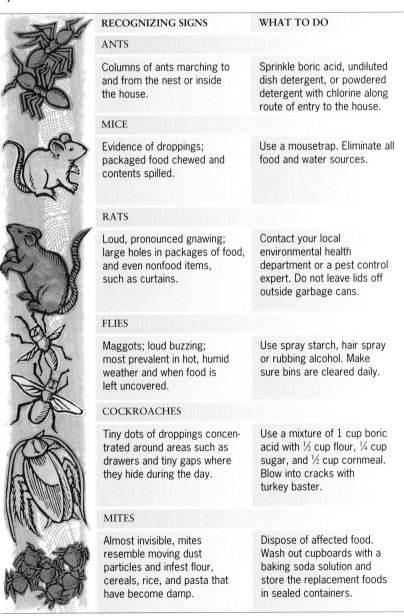

RECOGNIZING SIGNS	WHAT TO DO
ANTS	
Columns of ants marching to and from the nest or inside the house.	Sprinkle boric acid, undiluted dish detergent, or powdered detergent with chlorine along route of entry to the house.
MICE	
Evidence of droppings; packaged food chewed and contents spilled.	Use a mousetrap. Eliminate all food and water sources.
RATS	
Loud, pronounced gnawing; large holes in packages of food, and even nonfood items, such as curtains.	Contact your local environmental health department or a pest control expert. Do not leave lids off outside garbage cans.
FLIES	
Maggots; loud buzzing; most prevalent in hot, humid weather and when food is left uncovered.	Use spray starch, hair spray or rubbing alcohol. Make sure bins are cleared daily.
COCKROACHES	
Tiny dots of droppings concentrated around areas such as drawers and tiny gaps where they hide during the day.	Use a mixture of 1 cup boric acid with ½ cup flour, ¼ cup sugar, and ½ cup cornmeal. Blow into cracks with turkey baster.
MITES	
Almost invisible, mites resemble moving dust particles and infest flour, cereals, rice, and pasta that have become damp.	Dispose of affected food. Wash out cupboards with a baking soda solution and store the replacement foods in sealed containers.

145

Many foods—for example, chopped frozen vegetables—can be cooked without thawing first, but others need to be thoroughly defrosted, especially large pieces of meat and poultry. Defrosting ensures that the center of the food will be properly cooked. Thaw foods in the refrigerator, preferably on the bottom shelf or in cold water, but not at room temperature. When defrosting the freezer, put food in an ice chest to help keep it cold and prevent thawing before returning it to the freezer.

CHOOSING FRESH FOODS

When selecting fresh food, rely on your senses of touch, sight, smell, and taste. If you are in any doubt, do not buy it. Buy

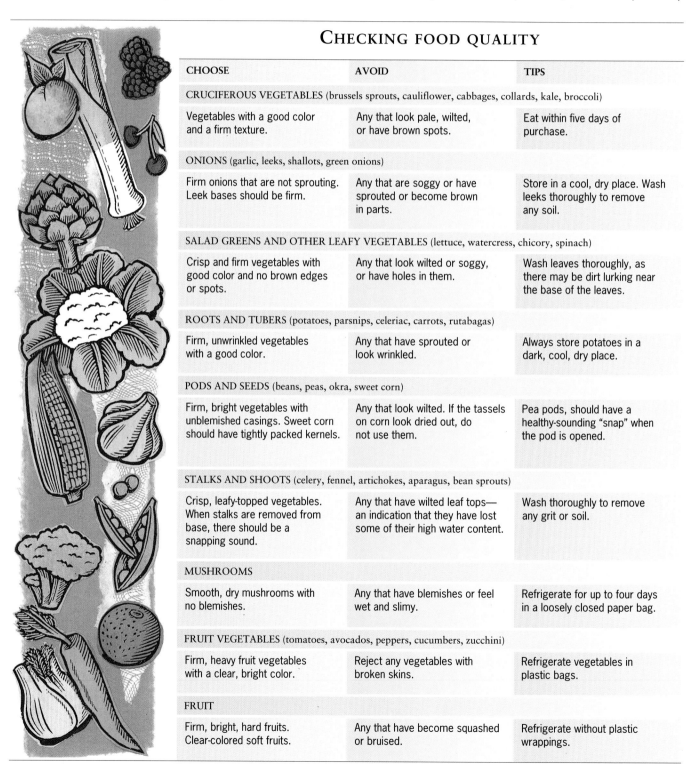

CHECKING FOOD QUALITY

CHOOSE	AVOID	TIPS
CRUCIFEROUS VEGETABLES (brussels sprouts, cauliflower, cabbages, collards, kale, broccoli)		
Vegetables with a good color and a firm texture.	Any that look pale, wilted, or have brown spots.	Eat within five days of purchase.
ONIONS (garlic, leeks, shallots, green onions)		
Firm onions that are not sprouting. Leek bases should be firm.	Any that are soggy or have sprouted or become brown in parts.	Store in a cool, dry place. Wash leeks thoroughly to remove any soil.
SALAD GREENS AND OTHER LEAFY VEGETABLES (lettuce, watercress, chicory, spinach)		
Crisp and firm vegetables with good color and no brown edges or spots.	Any that look wilted or soggy, or have holes in them.	Wash leaves thoroughly, as there may be dirt lurking near the base of the leaves.
ROOTS AND TUBERS (potatoes, parsnips, celeriac, carrots, rutabagas)		
Firm, unwrinkled vegetables with a good color.	Any that have sprouted or look wrinkled.	Always store potatoes in a dark, cool, dry place.
PODS AND SEEDS (beans, peas, okra, sweet corn)		
Firm, bright vegetables with unblemished casings. Sweet corn should have tightly packed kernels.	Any that look wilted. If the tassels on corn look dried out, do not use them.	Pea pods, should have a healthy-sounding "snap" when the pod is opened.
STALKS AND SHOOTS (celery, fennel, artichokes, aparagus, bean sprouts)		
Crisp, leafy-topped vegetables. When stalks are removed from base, there should be a snapping sound.	Any that have wilted leaf tops— an indication that they have lost some of their high water content.	Wash thoroughly to remove any grit or soil.
MUSHROOMS		
Smooth, dry mushrooms with no blemishes.	Any that have blemishes or feel wet and slimy.	Refrigerate for up to four days in a loosely closed paper bag.
FRUIT VEGETABLES (tomatoes, avocados, peppers, cucumbers, zucchini)		
Firm, heavy fruit vegetables with a clear, bright color.	Reject any vegetables with broken skins.	Refrigerate vegetables in plastic bags.
FRUIT		
Firm, bright, hard fruits. Clear-colored soft fruits.	Any that have become squashed or bruised.	Refrigerate without plastic wrappings.

foods only from reputable sources and avoid bargains, unless you intend to eat them on the day of purchase. Always take notice of the "use by" or "best before" dates for dairy products, meats, and eggs, and be ruthless about discarding food that has passed its peak. Buy fruits and vegetables often, preferably every two to three days.

When choosing seafood, let your nose be a guide; it should smell briny, without any hint of iodine or fishiness. Of the shellfish caught or farmed in American waters, most are available throughout the year, but some, such as oysters, cannot be eaten during the breeding season (May to August) because of poor quality. Crabs and lobsters sometimes

CHECKING FOOD QUALITY

CHOOSE	AVOID	TIPS
RED MEAT		
Beef with a deep red color and creamy-colored marble fat. Pork should be pale pink, with a close-grained texture and an even covering of fat. Choose plump joints of lamb with pliable skin and creamy-colored fat.	Beef that has an unnatural bright orange color or any pork with a grayish tinge and an oily fat covering. Avoid lamb with fat that is yellow and oily—this indicates an older piece of meat.	Beef, pork, and lamb can be kept for up to three days in the refrigerator. Pork can be kept for up to eight months and beef and lamb for up to a year in the freezer.
POULTRY		
Birds with a plump, well-rounded breast and skin that is firm and slightly creamy yellow in color.	Any bird that looks underfed or that has blemishes and bruises on its skin. Also avoid frozen birds that have frozen moisture in the package—this indicates it has thawed and been refrozen.	Refrigerate for up to two days and freeze for up to six months. Frozen birds must be defrosted thoroughly before cooking.
FISH		
Only the freshest fish. Choose a reputable fishmonger or supermarket and eat on the day of purchase. Fish should smell of the sea and have plenty of scales, and bright eyes. The gills should be red and the flesh firm. Frozen fish should be frozen solid, with no signs of water.	Any fish that has a strong fishy smell—an indication of high levels of bacteria—dull, opaque eyes, or slimy skin. The flesh of fresh fish bounces back immediately when pressed.	Fish should be refrigerated for only one day—in the coldest section—and frozen for up to six months. Oily fish spoils more easily: freeze only for up to three months. Fish that is bought frozen can be kept in the freezer and defrosted or cooked while frozen.
SHELLFISH		
Shellfish that is alive, to ensure freshness. Lobsters and crabs should move their legs when touched. Mussels and oysters should have tightly closed shells or, if opened, should close when tapped. Raw and cooked shrimp should be firm.	Mussels, clams, and oysters that open before cooking or that have failed to open after cooking. Avoid any shellfish with cracked or chipped shells.	Raw or cooked shrimp and cooked mussels can be frozen for up to a month. Cooked crab and lobster meat can be frozen for up to two months.
DAIRY PRODUCTS AND EGGS		
Products with a good, clear color and a fresh smell. Do not take any chances, particularly with eggs.	Cheese, butter, or milk that smells sour or rancid, and milk that has separated and looks watery. Do not buy eggs that are cracked.	If possible, eggs, milk, and yogurt should be used before the "sell by" date but should be okay for another week. Hard cheese can be refrigerated for up to a few months; soft cheese for only a week or two.

147

hibernate in very cold water and so are more abundant from April to Octo-ber. Scallops are also eaten during summer months, but mussel season is usually between September and March, when their meat is most plump. Purchase shellfish from markets that keep them well covered with ice or, in the case of lobsters, in aerated tanks.

STORING FOOD IN THE CUPBOARD

The foods in your cupboard are reliable standbys for the unexpected—visitors, illness, bad weather—because they have long shelf lives. No food lasts forever, however, and over time, food stored in the cupboard is just as susceptible to contamination and infestation as other foods. Regularly throw

FOODS FOR THE CUPBOARD

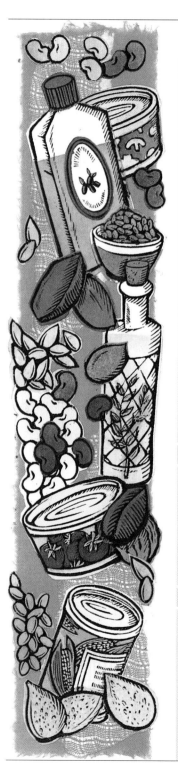

CHOOSING	USING	STORING
OILS AND FATS		
The best-quality general-purpose oil is high in unsaturated fat. Olive, canola, safflower, corn, or peanut oil should be chosen over lard, and butter. Cold-pressed (virgin) olive oil, extracted in the early stages of pressing, tastes better than oils that are extracted later. But it does not keep as well, so buy it in small quantities.	If you must deep-fry, use oil rather than fat, and preferably use the oil only once. Deep-frying changes oil because the fat of food fried in it dissolves into the oil. Gradual oxidation occurs, which is the early stage of rancidity. The oil will become darker and will foam on the surface when food is added.	Unopened oil in a glass bottle or can will keep for about a year. Once opened, most oils remain usable for about six months, provided you store them in a dark, cool place. (Hazelnut, walnut, and sesame oils should go in the refrigerator; they may congeal, but will liquefy when brought back to room temperature.) When oils become rancid, they should be thrown away.
DRIED BEANS, PEAS, AND LENTILS		
Make sure that beans are of a similar size and color. A bean loses its color as it gets older. Avoid any beans with cracks or tiny holes—an indication of possible insect damage.	Pick over beans, peas, and lentils and discard any stones or grit. Before cooking, most beans need to be soaked for about eight hours in cold water, and then rinsed to eliminate toxins. Follow package directions for cooking time.	Because they contain almost no fat, dried beans (except soybeans, which are high in fat) are ideal for storing in the cupboard, but they should be eaten within a year. Store in an airtight container in a cool, dry place.
NUTS AND SEEDS		
When buying nuts in their shells, try to buy them when they are at their peak of freshness, usually within a few weeks of harvesting in the fall. If a nut in its shell is old, it will rattle when you shake the shell	Most shelled nuts can be bought whole, chopped, ground, or slivered, and sometimes blanched, and require no further preparation.	Both nuts and seeds should be stored in a cool, dry place to preserve their oil content as long as possible. Store shelled nuts in airtight containers in the freezer. The store packaging is not ideal for long-term storage.
CANNED FOODS		
Avoid dented cans even if there are no signs of leakage or rust. Never use a can that has expanded and looks swollen. Also, look for canned foods with logos on the labels saying "reduced sodium" or "no salt added" or "no added sugar."	Once opened, the contents will deteriorate at the same rate as fresh cooked food. Never keep the contents in an open can, as this could lead to metal absorption.	Cans can be stored for four to five years, but check the "use by" date. If a can becomes rusty, dented, or has expanded, throw it away, as the food inside may be contaminated. Botulism—a form of food poisoning—can occur through home canning, if rules for canning methods and hygiene are not followed.

away any product that has exceeded its "use by" or "best before" date (the latter shows only the month and year for products that last longer than three months).

When restocking the cupboard, move older foods forward and place the new ones behind them so that the old foods are eaten first. Whenever you do this, make sure that you throw away any foods that are growing mold and any cans that have expanded or become rusty. To avoid insect infestations and contamination of food, clean the cupboard regularly with a mild disinfectant. Use a baking soda mixture, not ammonia or other household cleaners, so that there will be no danger of tainting the food.

FOODS FOR THE CUPBOARD

CHOOSING	USING	STORING
BREAKFAST CEREALS		
Choose cereals with a high fiber content. Avoid cartons that are torn or show signs of leakage. Sometimes they are accidentally slit by the store stacker opening the case with a sharp knife.	Instead of sugar, sprinkle pieces of chopped fruit, such as bananas, or dried fruit, such as raisins, onto the cereal.	Once opened, seal package with food clips or fold over the inner lining of the box. Store the box in a cool, dry place.
PASTA AND NOODLES		
Dried pasta and noodles should be brittle and smooth. Choose pasta made from whole-grain flour, which contains more fiber and zinc than refined flour.	Pasta and noodles require no preparation before cooking. Allow 4 oz of uncooked pasta per person and cook until "al dente" (offering some resistance to the teeth).	Dried pasta and noodles have a long shelf life when correctly stored because microorganisms rarely grow on them. Store them in an airtight container in a cool, dry place. Do not let them become exposed to moisture.
FLOUR		
Some of the vitamins and minerals lost in the refining process are added back to white flour by manufacturers, but it lacks fiber. Whole-grain flour contains about 10.8 g fiber per 3½ oz of flour. Avoid packages that are torn or show any signs of leakage.	If a recipe specifies sifted flour, pass it through a sieve before measuring it.	Keep flour in a cool, dry cupboard in an airtight container. (Whole-grain flour, which spoils more quickly, can be kept in the freezer.) Flour is vulnerable to flour mites, weevils, moths, and beetles. Check regularly and discard flour if you find signs of these pests, then wash down the cupboard with a mild disinfectant and scrupulously clean any containers the flour was kept in.
HERBS		
Buy only small amounts of dried herbs, as they will lose their pungency and flavor after a few months.	Dried herbs require no preparation before using. They are best used in slow-cooking dishes for a stronger flavor.	Keep dried herbs away from heat and light and store in airtight containers. Chopped fresh herbs can be frozen in ice cube trays filled with water.
SPICES		
Buy spices whole whenever possible, as they will retain their flavor and freshness much better.	Grind whole spices with a pestle and mortar or electric coffee grinder. If using whole spices in stews or soups, wrap in a muslin bag and tie the string to the pan handle for easy removal.	Keep in airtight jars, away from light and moisture. Many spices have long shelf lives, but keep an eye on the "use by" date and discard if exceeded. Stale spices tend to taste dry and dusty.

COOKING FOR BETTER HEALTH

Good cooking can enhance the flavor, appearance, smell, and texture of foods. But it should, at the same time, preserve nutritional content and prevent food poisoning.

Not only does food look and taste good when it is prepared well, but also the nutritional content is generally better, sometimes as much as three times greater than that of badly cooked food. Overexposure to air, too much added fat, excessive heat or cooking time, an unsuitable cooking method, and other variables can lower nutritional quality.

VEGETABLES

Vegetables contain enzymes that cause them to ripen and lose nutrients. Since light and air as well as heat accelerate enzyme activity, you should store vegetables in the refrigerator and use them as soon as possible after purchase. In order to preserve their goodness, do not wash, chop, slice, or cook vegetables until you are ready to eat them (except for leafy greens, which can be washed, spun dry, wrapped in paper towels, and refrigerated in plastic bags).

Wash vegetables before using, but do not soak them because water-soluble nutrients will leach into the water. Hold them briefly under cold running water and use a vegetable scrubbing brush to remove dirt from root vegetables like carrots. Peeled vegetables are less nutritious because some of their nutritional content lies in or just beneath the skin. If you do not want to eat them unpeeled, cook them in their skins, then peel them; fewer nutrients will be lost.

Retaining nutrients

When possible, avoid boiling vegetables because much of their nutritional goodness will disappear into the water. Instead, steam vegetables, cook them in a microwave, or stir-fry them using a minimum amount of water or oil. They should be cooked until crisp-tender (that is, they offer some resistance to the teeth, instead of being soft and soggy), so that they retain their color and texture. Do not use baking soda to preserve color; alkaline solutions destroy vitamins.

MICROWAVE COOKING

Microwaves cook by making the water molecules in food vibrate quickly, thereby generating heat. The microwaves penetrate to a depth of only 1 to 2 inches, so the heat spreads through the food by conduction—the food cooks from the outside inward.

Microwave ovens are quick and efficient and require very little liquid for cooking. They are ideal for steaming vegetables and fish, which lose the minimum amount of nutrients. But foods cook unevenly and there are "cold spots" and "hot spots." Using a rotating turntable and stirring helps food to cook more evenly. This approach also solves an important problem, because food-poisoning bacteria may grow in a cold spot. Always observe "standing" times after cooking as they are part of the overall cooking.

OVEN-BAKED POTATO
The hot, dry air in a conventional oven penetrates a potato slowly. After about 15 minutes, the center is still cool. It takes about an hour to cook through.

MICROWAVED POTATO
Although microwaving heats the potato through after about 5 minutes, standing time is needed for thorough cooking.

After 7 minutes	After 15 minutes
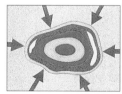	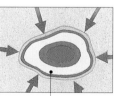

Heat slowly spreads through conduction.

After 1½ minutes	After 5 minutes
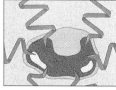	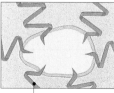

Vibrating molecules generate heat, which spreads through conduction.

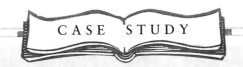

A Vegetarian in the Family

In a household where meat is the principal source of protein, the sudden decision of one member to switch to a vegetarian diet can throw the family cook into a quandary. Where will the vegetarian get the protein he or she needs for a healthy, well-balanced diet? And does this mean that every meal will require the preparation of two separate menus?

Sixteen-year-old Sarah, who has always been interested in environmental issues, announces to her parents that she has become a vegetarian. Her mother, Liz, is not entirely surprised. Although Liz is an enthusiastic cook with a large collection of cookbooks, her meals have always been meat-oriented: beef and lamb stews, chops, and a traditional roast on Sundays. Food shopping routinely ends with a trip to the local delicatessen for the pâtés, salamis, and hams that the family favors for sandwiches and snacks. And although she wants to keep Sarah happy, Liz cannot take on too much extra catering: She teaches at a nursery school and is studying part-time for a degree.

WHAT SHOULD LIZ DO?

Liz should start by investigating nonmeat sources of protein and iron to make sure that Sarah does not suffer deficiencies in her diet. Once she explores her local health food shop and scans through a few vegetarian cookbooks, she will be reassured about the wide range of alternative protein sources, not only the predictable options of dairy products but also combinations of grains and beans that provide as much protein as one of her husband's steaks. If she does not object to convenience foods, she can buy a wide selection of vegetarian pies based on tofu or beans, and meatless sausages made with textured vegetable protein, known as TVP.

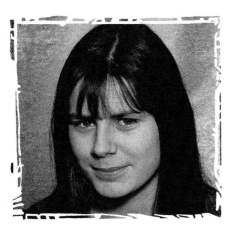

COOKING CONCERNS
Many vegetarian dishes take longer to prepare if made from scratch.

HEALTH CONCERNS
Lack of iron in the diet will lead to anemia, which results in tiredness, weakness, and shortness of breath.

A VARIED DIET
If a vegetarian diet is not well thought out, it may become as unbalanced as that of many meat eaters.

Action Plan

HEALTH
Provide whole-wheat cereals and dark green vegetables, which are quite high in iron. Offer orange juice with meals to increase iron absorption from nonmeat foods.

A VARIED DIET
Experiment with new foods and dishes. For packed lunches and after-school snacks, try chickpea-based hummus and pâtés made of spinach, mushrooms, and carrots.

COOKING METHODS
Prepare dishes like vegetable soups, stews, and casseroles that can be frozen then reheated.

HOW THINGS TURN OUT FOR LIZ AND SARAH

Liz was happy to see that Sarah's vegetarianism has led her to become more adventurous in her eating habits and even inspired her to try her hand at cooking for herself and her parents. Four nights a week, Liz still cooks a meat dish for herself and her husband, Neil, and provides a vegetarian alternative for Sarah. But on these nights, she wishes that Sarah would refrain from criticizing her parents' carnivorous appetites while at the table.

Cooking vegetables whole or in large pieces helps to preserve their nutritional content. There is less surface area exposed to the air and so less nutrients will be oxidized. Reserve the water after cooking vegetables and use it for making soups or gravies. Cooking vegetables in a wok (stir-frying) is a good way to preserve their nutrients because the vegetables are coated with a small amount of oil and are in con-

METHODS OF COOKING

COOKING METHOD	BENEFITS	DISADVANTAGES
DEEP-FRYING		
Quick cooking in boiling fat.	Some vitamins retained.	Fat content of foods increased.
DRY FRYING		
Fat-free frying.	No fat added; good retention of vitamins and minerals.	Suitable only for foods containing some natural fat.
STIR-FRYING (WOK COOKING)		
Quick method of cooking over high heat.	Crisp look and taste. Little fat is needed. Minimal vitamin loss.	High in salt if too much soy sauce is used.
MICROWAVING		
Cooking in a microwave oven (see page 150).	Minimal vitamin loss.	Uneven cooking, with "cold" and "hot" spots in food.
BRAISING AND STEWING		
Slow cooking in liquid over several hours.	Flavor and texture of tough cuts of meat improved.	Vitamins leach into liquid, but retention in stewing is better than in roasting.
GRILLING AND BROILING		
Quick cooking with dry heat.	No fat added; vitamins and minerals lost to drippings.	Formation of carcinogens may be induced by charcoal or open-flame grilling of meats.
BOILING		
Cooking in large amounts of water.	Improved texture of tough vegetables.	Some vitamins lost to liquid.
POACHING		
Simmering in a little liquid.	No added fat.	Some vitamin loss.
STEAMING		
Cooking over steam that is converted from a little water.	Preserves most nutrients and flavor.	Careful watching of cooking time needed to prevent overcooking.
ROASTING		
Cooking with intense, dry heat.	Succulent meat; some retention of vitamins in vegetables.	Vitamin loss. Fat added to meat with the basting.
POT ROASTING		
Slow baking in covered dish.	No added fat.	Some vitamin loss.
PRESSURE COOKING		
Quick cooking at high temperature with minimal water.	Most vitamins and minerals preserved.	Timing difficult to control, which may cause overcooking.

tact with heat for a minimum amount of time. Once cooked, vegetables should be served and eaten as soon as possible because they will begin to lose their nutritional content if allowed to stand.

MEAT

A rich source of protein, B vitamins, and minerals, meat can be a valuable part of a healthy diet. Protein does not diminish during cooking, and although vitamins and some minerals may leach into the cooking medium, you can use it to make soups, sauces, and gravies.

Most meats, lamb and beef in particular, are high in saturated fat. Avoid excess fat by purchasing lean cuts of meat, such as round or sirloin tip. Make sure that you trim off all external fat. Meats that have been trimmed of fat require less cooking time than fatty meats. Therefore, reduce the normal cooking time by about 20 percent. Rare meat will be more tender, but always make sure that it is not undercooked (see box, below).

Use fat-free cooking methods, such as steaming, braising, and grilling, as often as possible. When making a stew, skim the fat off the top at regular intervals. Avoid frying meats, but if you do fry them, use olive or canola oil, both of which are high in monounsaturated fats, instead of butter. Dry fry fatty meats such as ground beef in nonstick pans, then drain off the fat that is released during cooking. Before roasting meat, place it on a rack inside the roasting pan. This allows the fat to drip below the meat when it is cooking.

POULTRY

Chicken is an excellent source of protein and contains less fat than some meats, especially when the skin is removed. Frozen chicken must be thoroughly defrosted. Before cooking, rinse the skin and the cavity and pat dry with paper towels. Always marinate chicken (and meat) in the refrigerator, not at room temperature.

Because of the risk of salmonella poisoning, poultry must never be undercooked. Place fatty birds like duck and goose on a rack in a roasting pan, then prick the skin before roasting. This allows fat to escape. Chicken is extremely versatile and can be cooked in a variety of healthy ways, such as stir-frying, baking in foil or parchment paper, or poaching (see page 141).

FISH AND SHELLFISH

An especially healthful food, fish is high in protein and relatively low in fat. Moreover, certain fish, such as salmon, trout, tuna,

TESTING FOR DONENESS

Overcooked meat is dry and stringy. Eating undercooked meat and poultry, however, can be dangerous. Animal foods are particularly vulnerable to food-poisoning bacteria, which are killed if food is thoroughly cooked.

A reliable method of measuring the doneness of meat is to use a meat thermometer. It should be inserted into the thickest part of the flesh. Do not let it touch the bone, which conducts heat and will be hotter than the surrounding meat.

For rare beef and lamb, the meat thermometer will show 140°F; for medium it will show 160°F.

It is essential that pork be well cooked because it may be contaminated with a parasite that causes the disease trichinosis. When pork is well cooked, it will give a reading of 170°F.

Cooking poultry thoroughly will protect you against poisoning by salmonella bacteria. To check the doneness of a chicken, turkey, duck, or goose, insert a poultry thermometer into the thickest part of the meat away from the bone. For a whole bird, the thermometer will read 180°F; for breast, thigh, and wing pieces, it will read 170°F.

Another more commonly used way of testing poultry for doneness is to stick a skewer into the fleshiest part of the thigh and then let the juices run out. They should be clear, not pink. Alternatively, raise the whole bird with a two-pronged fork and check the juices as they run out of the cavity into the dish.

Fish is cooked when the eyes are opaque and the flesh flakes easily when tested with a fork.

153

Dangerous microbes

If a food is contaminated with large numbers of bacteria, such as salmonella or listeria, it will cause food poisoning. But campylobacteria are dangerous even in small numbers.

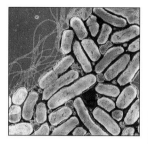

SALMONELLA BACTERIA
Infants, the elderly, and people with weakened immune systems, such as cancer sufferers, are particularly vulnerable to salmonella poisoning.

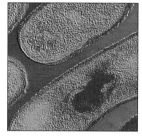

LISTERIA
Pregnant women should avoid soft cheeses and undercooked meat, as these bacteria can be fatal for unborn babies.

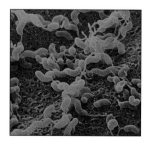

CAMPYLOBACTERIA
The bacteria live in animals and wild birds and can be picked up by humans touching animals or raw poultry.

and mackerel, are rich in omega-3 fatty acids that may help to prevent heart disease. Shellfish are important sources of minerals, such as zinc.

All fish should be scaled and gutted before cooking. Rinse fish under cold running water and pat dry with paper towels. Steaming, microwaving, grilling, and poaching will retain the fish's moisture without adding much fat. Fish cooks perfectly in a microwave oven, but slash the skin to prevent pressure building up and splitting the fish. Baking fish in foil or parchment paper will help to retain flavor (see page 141).

Scrub mollusks under cold running water and discard any that stay open when tapped lightly. Shellfish need to be boiled for only a few minutes. Throw away any clams, mussels, or oysters that have not opened after cooking.

FOOD POISONING

Despite the advances in food processing and distribution that have helped to make food fresher and healthier, food poisoning is on the increase. In England and Wales, the increase of reported cases has been dramatic, rising from 14,253 in 1982 to 63,347 in 1992. In the United States in 1978, there were 28,881 cases of food poisoning caused by the salmonella bacteria reported to the Centers for Disease Control and Prevention (CDC). By 1987, the number of reported cases had almost doubled. The CDC estimates the number of people who are actually affected by food poisoning to be even higher.

Careless handling of food before and after cooking and improper heating causes bacteria to grow at an alarming rate. But food poisoning is preventable with careful preparation, storage, and cooking.

Causes of food poisoning

Bacteria are single-cell organisms that are invisible to the naked eye. With suitable temperatures, bacteria can double their numbers in 20 minutes. Bacteria are transferred to humans either from food—poultry and eggs are typical examples of salmonella carriers—or from the excrement of infected people or animals.

The most common disease-producing bacteria belong to the salmonella and campylobacter groups. They can multiply with tremendous rapidity in the intestines

CONTROLLING BACTERIA

Meat, poultry, and eggs all harbor bacteria that can be destroyed when heated properly. If a food is kept at a temperature within the "danger zone," however, it may cause serious illness when eaten.

▶ *Cooking temperatures (165°F and up) destroy most bacteria. The higher the temperature, the less time needed to kill bacteria.*

▶ *Warming temperatures (140°F to 165°F) prevent the growth of bacteria, but they still survive.*

▶ *Bacteria grow rapidly and produce toxins in temperatures between 60°F and 120°F.*

▶ *Cold temperatures (32°F to 42°F) allow the slow growth of bacteria.*

▶ *Freezing temperatures (0°F to 14°F) prevent the growth of bacteria but do not kill them.*

and cause widespread inflammation. Some types of bacteria—for example, *Staphylococcus aureus* and *Clostridium botulinum*—produce toxins that cause food poisoning upon ingestion.

Symptoms

Nausea, diarrhea, vomiting, and stomach pain are common symptoms of food poisoning. Severe cases may also include shock and collapse. Botulism toxin, however, has a different set of symptoms that affect the central nervous system and cause visual disturbances, problems with speech, muscle paralysis, and vomiting.

Viruses do not multiply in foods, but they do contaminate certain foods from seabeds polluted by untreated sewage. There can be serious consequences from eating raw shellfish and raw fish (sushi). Always buy fish from a reputable supplier.

What to do for food poisoning

With the exception of poisoning from mushrooms, from *E. coli* 0157:H7, or botulism poisoning, episodes of food poisoning, although unpleasant, are rarely fatal. Someone who is suffering from food poisoning should avoid solid foods until the symptoms clear up and drink plenty of fluids to rehydrate the body. Babies, toddlers, and elderly people are particularly at risk from dehydration. An oral rehydration solution is the best way to treat this conditin. You can buy one from a pharmacist or make your own (1 teaspoon of salt and 8 teaspoons of sugar in 1 quart of water). Lethargy and weakness are common until the poisoning clears the body, so rest will be necessary.

For severe vomiting and diarrhea or if the affected person collapses, seek medical help immediately. The sufferer may be required to provide a fecal sample so that it can be analyzed to identify the cause. If you have kept a sample of the food responsible, it should also be sent away for analysis. If a restaurant is responsible, inform your local health department.

FOOD POISONING SYMPTOMS

Reactions to food poisoning can vary, but they are mostly dependent on the extent of the contamination to which the food has been expoʻsed. The most common causes of food poisoning are shown in the chart below.

SYMPTOMS	ONSET	AFFECTED FOODS
E. COLI 0157:H7 ✳✳		
Abdominal cramps, diarrhea, vomiting, low-grade fever.	3 to 4 days.	Undercooked hamburger or roast beef, unpasteurized milk.
CHEMICAL POISONING ✳✳		
Diarrhea, vomiting.	Within 30 minutes.	Seafood from polluted water.
STAPHYLOCOCCAL TOXINS ✳✳✳		
Vomiting, nausea, diarrhea, abdominal cramps.	1 to 6 hours.	Meat, poultry, egg, and dairy dishes.
CLOSTRIDIUM PERFRINGENS ✳✳✳		
Diarrhea, abdominal cramps.	6 to 12 hours.	Meat, gravies, stuffing.
BOTULISM (CLOSTRIDIUM BOTULINUM) ✳✳		
Slurred speech, blurred vision, paralysis. Death can occur from respiratory failure.	12 to 36 hours.	Improperly canned foods, foods contaminated by flies.
SALMONELLA ORGANISMS ✳		
Diarrhea, vomiting, fever, abdominal cramps, headache.	8 to 48 hours.	Poultry, eggs, raw meat, dairy products, shellfish.
VIRUSES (HEPATITIS A) ✳✳		
Diarrhea, vomiting, fever, jaundice. Severe cases can be fatal.	12 to 48 hours.	Contaminated seafood, especially raw shellfish.
SHIGELLA ORGANISMS ✳✳✳		
Abdominal cramps, fever, diarrhea.	2 to 3 days.	Dairy products, tuna, poultry, potato salad.
CAMPYLOBACTERIA ✳✳✳		
Abdominal cramps, fever, diarrhea, sometimes bloody stools.	2 to 6 days.	Meat, poultry, milk.
LISTERIA MONOCYTOGENES ✳✳		
Headache, nausea, fever.	7 to 30 days.	Soft cheese, seafood, pâté.

✳ See your doctor if symptoms persist　　✳✳ Seek medical help immediately　　✳✳✳ Rest and take plenty of fluids

Natural toxins
A wide variety of foods contain natural poisons that are harmful only if eaten in large amounts. Small fish and shellfish feeding off algae may also ingest algal toxins. These accumulate in their flesh and in the flesh of larger predator fish such as snapper and sea bass. The toxins can reach levels that are poisonous to humans. Ciguatera poisoning, which is caused by ingesting fish contaminated with algal toxins, occurs occasionally in the United States; the symptoms include cramps and numb and tingling lips. Shellfish are regularly monitored for toxins in the United States.

The potato also harbors a natural toxin, solanin, which is usually present in low levels. High levels of this toxin are found in the green parts of potatoes, in sprouted potatoes, and in potatoes exposed to light. Because this toxin is not destroyed by cooking, the green parts must be discarded.

CONVERSION TABLES

The tables below provide rounded-out equivalents in weight for imperial and metric measurements. Following one or the other when preparing a recipe should yield successful results. However, it is important to stick to one or the other system and not switch within a recipe, otherwise the proportions will change slightly.

MEASURING CUPS

In the United States, the standard measuring tool is the 8-ounce cup. Volume measurement is used for both liquid and dry ingredients. In other countries, ingredients are measured by weight. Below is a selection of foods and their equivalent metric and imperial weights.

Measuring cups for ¼, ⅓, ½, and 1 cup are used for dry ingredients.

Teaspoons and tablespoons can be used for both liquid and dry ingredients.

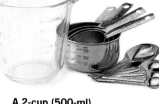

A 2-cup (500-ml) measuring cup is useful when measuring large amounts. Make sure you check the volume of liquid at eye level.

White rice 1 cup = 6 oz (170 g)

White beans 1 cup = 8 oz (225 g)

Sifted flour and cocoa 1 cup = 4 oz (115 g)

Butter 1 stick = 4 oz (115 g)

Parmesan cheese 1 cup, grated = 4 oz (115 g)

Sugar (granulated) 1 cup = 8 oz (225 g)

Red kidney beans 8 oz (225 g)

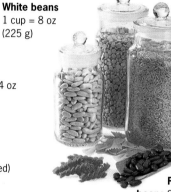

WEIGHT CHART

DRY MEASURES		LIQUID MEASURES	
IMPERIAL	METRIC	IMPERIAL	METRIC
½ oz	15 g	1 teaspoon	5 ml
1 oz	30 g	1 tablespoon	15 ml
1½ oz	45 g	2 tbsp	30 ml
2 oz	60 g	4 tbsp	60 ml
2½ oz	70 g	3 fl oz	85 ml
3 oz	85 g	4 fl oz	115 ml
3½ oz	100 g	5 fl oz	150 ml
4 oz	115 g	6 fl oz	175 ml
5 oz	140 g	7 fl oz	200 ml
6 oz	170 g	8 fl oz	225 ml
7 oz	200 g	10 fl oz	285 ml
8 oz	225 g	12 fl oz	340 ml
10 oz	275 g	15 fl oz	425 ml
12 oz	340 g	16 fl oz	450 ml
16 oz (1 lb)	450 g	1 pint	570 ml

TEMPERATURES

OVEN TEMPERATURES		
°F	°C	DIAL MARK
150	80	Keep warm
175	90	Keep warm
200	100	Keep warm
225	110	Low
250	120	Low
275	140	Low
300	150	Low
325	160	Medium
350	180	Medium
375	190	Medium
400	200	Hot
425	220	Hot
450	230	Hot
475	240	Very hot
500	250	Very hot

INDEX

ACKNOWLEDGEMENTS

Carroll & Brown Limited
would like to thank
Dr Frazer Anderson
   Musculoskeletal Unit,
   Freeman Hospital,
   Newcastle upon Tyne

Ellen Dupont
Melanie Hulse
Sue Mimms

British Heart Foundation
Child Growth Foundation
The Coeliac Society
Ealing Active Leisure
   London Borough of Ealing
The Shellfish Association
The Vegetarian Society
Zenith International Ltd

Photograph sources
8 Popperfoto
9 Popperfoto
10 Range Pictures
11 Zefa
28 Niall McInerney
33 Matt Meadows/Peter Arnold
Inc/SPL
44 David Parker/SPL
54 National Library of Medicine/SPL
66 (Top left) Image Bank/David de
Lossy, (Bottom left) Eric Grave/SPL,
(Bottom right) National Medical
Slide Bank
69 (Left and right) Professor P. Motta,
Department of Anatomy, University
"La Sapienza", Rome/SPL
80 Pictures Colour Library
91 (Top) Image Bank/Gerald
Brimacombe, (Bottom) Mike
Newton/The Robert Harding
Picture Library
102 CNRI/SPL
110 CNRI/SPL
114 Pictures Colour Library
124 Peter Tizzard
135 (Top) Giraudon/Bridgeman Art
Library, (Bottom) Niall McInerney
154 (Top) A.B. Dowsett/SPL, (Centre)
Institut Pasteur/CNRI/SPL, (Bottom)
Moredun Animal Health Ltd/SPL

Illustrators
Joanna Cameron
Jane Craddock-Watson
Eugene Fleury
John Geary
Christine Pilsworth
Paul Williams
Angela Wood

Charts
Clive Bruton
Lee Maunder
Nick Roland

Photographic assistance
Nick Allen
Ian Body
Alex Hansen
Sid Sideris

Picture researcher
Sandra Schneider

Food preparation
Maddalena Bastianelli
Eric Treuille

Research
Laura Price

Index
Madeline Weston

Note
Imperial measures are given throughout
except when calculating measures of
nutrients, which are given in metric.